i

'D' tales

Volume 1

5.5 Readings

Publishing Stories by Diabetics, for Diabetics

Dedicated to the
Half Billion
Diabetics
Worldwide

ISBN - 13: 978-1519434630
ISBN - 10: 1519434634
Third Edition: November 2015
Edited by Mia Esposa
Published by *5.5 Readings*

For
The love of my life
My best friend, my wife
Suzi

With Love & Thanks

These special people have my undying gratitude and
affection for their influences, odd perspectives and
laughter;
Mia Esposa, Roberta Green, Dr. David Johnstone,
Dr. Jim Bjork, Dr. Richard Bernstein,
L.J. Savage, Carlos Gardeazabal, Scott McKay,
Irene Whittem, Mike Priorello, Debbie Watson,
Gary and Ainsley Driver,
Magdalene Sinthern, Rolf Imwinkelreid,
Melody Richardson, Wendie Donabie,
members of the Bracebridge and Baysville
writing circles,
The Dream Catchers Writing Club in Huntsville,
and of course
The Boys:
Craig Scollick, Udo Wadien, &
Barry 'Fishy' Miller.

iv

Table of Contents

i

Chapter 1

The Test

The familiar squeak of the third step woke me from a light sleep. I froze, listening as slippers padded up the remaining carpeted steps. Mom was coming to wake me. I kept my eyes shut, my breathing slow and deep, pretending to be asleep. I felt the air pressure change when she entered my room. As she stepped closer, I could smell mom. My left cheek grew warmer, just before she gave me a light loving kiss and softly whispered, "Good morning sweet heart, rise and shine." I rolled over slowly, blinked open my eyes and smiled broadly. "Mmmorning mom," it felt good to be home. I stretched out full length like a cat, luxuriating in the comfort of my own bed, in my own room. I'd just spent the Christmas holidays in a metal and plastic bed at Sick Kids hospital. This was only my third morning back home since I got diabetes, but the first morning I was going to perform magic by myself.

Okay, so it wasn't actually magic, just a simple chemical experiment to gauge my blood sugars, but to a four year old boy, it was magic. Yesterday my mom had performed the magic right before my eyes and called it 'the test'. We were standing in the main floor two piece bathroom of our new house. She'd handed me a yellow plastic cup and told me to pee into it, then turned away to set up the rest of the experiment on the sink counter. I immediately did as she said, opening my pajama fly, taking out my pee pee and I swear, trying my best to hit the tiny yellow cup while holding my fly open and aiming with one hand. No easy trick for someone who, until very recently, had been pulling down his pants and squatting to do all his business. I ended up waving the cup around trying to catch my wandering pee stream. It moved closer, then farther, left and right like it had a mind of its own. It was frustrating and funny at the same time.

My mother totally disagreed. Turning around to take the cup, but seeing me peeing all over the bathroom floor, she screamed. I jumped and tensed up which caused my pee stream to arc way past the ½ full cup in my hand and onto her house coat. Quick as lightning she grabbed me by the shoulders, spun me round and stood me in front of the toilet. To my mom's dismay I kept peeing until facing the toilet, then trickled to a stop on the seat.

My mom had stared at me, "Did you do that on purpose?" I'd shrugged not understanding what she was talking about. I was way too scared to pee anymore and hoped there was enough in the cup for the test. My mom closed her eyes, inhaled deeply and exhaled slowly, three times. "Look, you're a big boy now," she'd started, "I know it's too late today, but tomorrow, and forever more, face the toilet and lift the seat before you start peeing. If you can't remember that, then at least don't pee on the seat. I don't want to have to clean this bathroom *every* day, okay?" I nodded and closed my fly.

Mom took the yellow cup from me and placed it on the counter with some other strange equipment.

"Now pay attention you're going to have to do this yourself one day," she said holding up a clear glass tube between her thumb and forefinger,
"This is a test tube."
"Tess tupe," I parroted as best I could.
She put it down and picked up a much smaller clear glass tube with a brown rubber ball at one end she said,
"This is an eyedropper."
"Eyedobba," I said nodding fascinated by the shiny new toys and the cautious way mom was handling them.

Holding the rubber ball between thumb and forefinger, my mom stuck the tapered end of the eyedropper into my pee. She squeezed the rubber ball and bubbles appeared. It was like blowing bubbles in my milk through a straw. Then awestruck, I watched as my pee climbed up inside the eyedropper. "How the heck?" I wondered, but before I could ask, she put the eyedropper's tip into the open end of the test tube, squeezed the ball and counted three drops into it.

"That's all?" I asked staring at the hard fought, half full cup of pee.

"Yes dear, just three drops," she said squirting the remaining pee in the eyedropper back into the yellow cup. "Five of water," she added, drawing water up into the eyedropper from a white plastic cup she'd filled earlier. She counted the water drops into the test tube then stood the eyedropper up in the cup of water.

Mom picked up a tablet from the counter, she'd taken it from a metal tube earlier. A tube with pictures of a skull and a skeleton hand. The tablet was white with blue speckles. She looked at me with her serious face and holding up the tablet said, "This is very dangerous, don't touch it with wet hands. Don't put it on a wet counter. And for God's sake don't put it in your mouth." With those warnings she plopped the tablet into the test tube.

At first nothing happened, the tablet just sat in the liquid at the bottom of the test tube. But a second later, tiny bubbles appeared on the tablet's surface just before it flipped over, then again and again, faster and faster. Bubbles became foam that began to climb up the clear sides of the test tube. A foul odor made my nose wrinkle, and I heard a sizzling & crackling noise come from the volatile concoction. "It's getting hot," said my mother. Bubbles crawled over each other in a desperate race to the top of the test tube.

Then, just before the angry foam escaped the test tube and burned my mother's fingers, the sizzling sound died down. The bubbles began to rupture and recede down the glass wall until they had completely disappeared. I stared at the test tube in wonder. The mostly transparent pee and water mixture was gone. In it's place was an opaque, bright turquoise liquid. My jaw dropped. "Let me try," I screamed, grabbing for the still hot test tube with both hands. Good thing my mom had developed cat like reflexes raising me. She lifted the test tube out of my reach the second she saw movement.

My mom reluctantly agreed to show me how to do the experiment after the test tube had cooled. While we waited she showed me how to color in the log book with my daily test results.

The color left in the test tube indicated the amount of sugar in my pee.

Blue, or 'Negative' meant no sugar. That was a 'good' result.

Turquoise or 'Trace' meant a tiny amount of sugar. Also considered a 'good' result.

Green or 1+ meant small amounts sugar. Not 'good', but not 'bad'.

Yellow or 2+, significant amounts of sugar. This was where 'bad' started.

Orange or 3+, excessive amounts of sugar. Really 'bad'.

Brown or 4+, dangerous amounts of sugar. Evil 'bad'

We repeated the test, with me doing most of the heavy lifting this time. Mom still had to help me along, but only once or twice.

Today, I was going to do the experiment all by myself. "Like a little scientist in his Lab," my dad had said last night before bed. He made being a scientist sound cool. After waking me, mom heard my six month old baby brother Steven start crying. She went back downstairs to look after him and get breakfast ready.

I threw back the covers, slipped on my slippers and raced downstairs to the two pc. bathroom on the main floor of our side split. The Lab as dad had called it. As I flashed by my mom feeding Steven in the kitchen, she said, "Show me the test tube before you empty it out okay? Are you sure you can do the test?"

"Sure mom," I said answering both questions at once, then ducked into my lab. The counter was empty. Mom hadn't taken the test tube and stuff out of the cupboard above the sink for me. I tried to reach the cupboard door's handle, but even on tiptoes and stretching as far as I could, it was just out of reach. I couldn't bring myself to call my mom already.

Putting my hands on the counter either side of the sink I hopped up, but my feet banged into the cupboard doors below the sink and an instant later my mom yelled out, "Are you all right in there, you need some help?"

I was embarrassed at making so much noise and giving away my dilemma, but I was also mad at my mom for not getting stuff ready for me. "I'm fine mom, just kicked the cupboard by accident, sorry," I said with a grunt as I got my left knee up onto the counter, then the right one. To open the cupboard doors enough to get my test tube and stuff I had to lean back balancing on my knees while holding the door open and reaching inside. I managed to get what I needed onto the counter top and jumped down quietly.

This time I remembered to stand in front of the toilet before trying to pee into the cup. I forgot to lift the lid, but remembered not to pee on it. I filled the cup only enough to do the test. The rest I peed into the toilet, closer and closer to the lid's edge. I wanted to see how close I could get without wetting the seat. I got to within a half inch before drops began to splash onto the seat. That wasn't really peeing on the seat, surely mom wouldn't notice, so I left it, promising to try harder tomorrow.

Resisting the urge to flush, like my parents had just trained me to, I turned around and put the yellow cup on the sink counter. Then I stretched over the counter to turn on the cold water and half fill the water cup. Taking a deep breath, I carefully picked up the test tube between my thumb and forefinger of one hand. Then picked up the eyedropper by its rubber ball with my other hand. The experiment had begun.

I stuck the glass end of the eyedropper into the cup of pee and waited. Nothing happened. My pee didn't slide up the glass tube like it had for my mother yesterday. I was doing something wrong, but it was still too soon to call for help. Then I remembered, and squeezing the rubber ball, made bubbles in my pee. When I slowly released the pressure on the rubber ball the pee raced up the eyedropper almost to the rubber ball. I was doing it.

My hands shook as I moved the eyedropper from the cup to the top of the test tube. I had problems holding it over the open end while squeezing the rubber ball gently enough so only... wait a second, was it three drops or five drops. Knowing this part was important to get right. I was about to give in and call mom, when I remembered that three came before five when I counted to ten.

I held my breath until I finished counting then sighed and squirted the remaining pee all over the pee cup. I swear, not a drop went in. I wiped it up with a Kleenex then carried on. Filling the eyedropper with water I counted six drops, the first one had missed the test tube entirely.

Then I reached for a tablet. The tube of tablets still had it's cap on. I tried but couldn't open it with one hand. I leaned the test tube against the lip of the sink so it wouldn't spill, but as soon as I let go of the test tube it rolled off the lip, spilling the pee/water all over the counter.

I didn't know where to start, clean up the pee or open the tube and get a tablet out. Either way I was going to have to start over, so I pulled out another Kleenex and wiped the counter and the test tube. I had just picked up the test tube when my mom called out, "David, how's it going in there? You need some help?" "No mom, I'm almost done, don't bug me," I called back angry with myself for not doing it right the first time.

Taking another deep breath, I filled the eyedropper with pee again, then remembered I hadn't taken a tablet out of the tube yet. I put down the eyedropper and opened the tube. I cupped one hand and tipped the tube so a tablet would roll out into it. All the tablets poured into my hand and overflowed onto the counter. A couple even rolled off the counter onto the floor. I scrambled to gather them up and forced them back into the tube, even the broken ones.

Finally I ended up with just one tablet on the counter. I picked up the eyedropper and test tube then continued the experiment. Once the drops were counted into the test tube, I picked up the dangerous tablet and popped it into the mix.

It started flipping and sizzling and the bubbles raced up the test tube walls. I held it up to watch closer as the tablet dissolved away and the liquid changed color. A dull brown liquid remained when the bubbles had disappeared. I didn't like that color and down right hated it when I matched it to the chart in the front of my log book. It was '4 +'. The worst result there was. I'd failed my first test.

I didn't want to show my mom that result. It was embarrassing. I'd always been the strongest, tallest, happiest kid out of all the kids I knew. I'd always done well on tests. How had I messed up?

When I finally got up the nerve to show my mom the bad result she just shook her head and sighed.

Not so bad, I thought, seizing the tiny victory and running back to the bathroom to finish up. I dumped the test tube's toxic chemicals, pee and water into the toilet and finally flushed.

Over the next month, whenever a 'good' result, like a negative or trace popped up, mom would sigh, as if relieved, smile at me and say, "Good boy." Honey sweet words to my ears. But when I got a 'bad' result and the liquid turned brown, and it turned brown a lot, she didn't smile. She'd look down, shake her head and sigh, "David?" Her tone asked why I wasn't trying harder, while suggesting that I could do better, had done better, and had to do better.

I didn't know what else to do. I stuck to my diet, ran around outside with the other normal kids like I was supposed to. Plus I was giving my own needle now and hadn't missed a day. What more *could* I do?

I tried lying, by calling out slightly better results from the bathroom, a 3 + instead of the 4 +, but mom wanted to see the test tube every morning and always saw a worse color than me.

One morning, I was extra sleepy when I did my test, accidentally adding six drops of water instead of five. I realized the miscount, but finished the test out of curiosity. 2+ was the result. Having been told my life depended on doing the test right, I retested for the first time, paying closer attention to the exact number of drops used.

The second 'true' result was 4+. *Wow, just one extra drop of water made the result so much better. What happens if I add two extra drops?* I pondered, and a scientist was born.

That morning I conducted three secret unsanctioned experiments. Working as fast as I could so Mom wouldn't notice how much longer than usual my test was taking. Through trial and error, I discovered that a 4+ could be changed into a Negative with just three extra drops of water.

Out of a misplaced desire to please my parents, and a child's malleable ethics, I changed the test. I was scared and excited when I showed my mom the first doctored test tube. Would she notice the higher liquid level in the test tube from the extra drops? What would be my punishment? Would they stop loving me? Think less of me? Mom barely glanced at the test tube, said, "Good boy," and went on making breakfast while holding Steven in one arm.

I'd done it. Mom had been fooled. It was the most thrilling moment of my short life. I felt empowered, in control. I'd never be a 'bad' boy again. I stood there a moment longer than usual. What do I do now? I fought the urge to jump up and down and boast how I'd fooled her. I hadn't completely believed I'd get away with the crime. Now all I had to do to make my parents happy was perform a second altered test whenever I got a bad result. I turned around and went back to my lab to clean up and record the first lie in my logbook.

According to the next week's test results, I was cured, blue in the tube every morning. My logbook had so many blue squares in a row they made a blue line that ran down the whole page.

Mom smiled and nodded at my great results for the first three or four mornings, but she was no fool. That many perfect test results in a row wasn't normal for me and that made her spider sense tingle.

Although dubious of my fantastic results, she couldn't figure out how I was doing it. She saw the test tube evidence daily. One morning when I held up yet another blue test tube, she looked me in the eye and asked me how? I blushed and shrugged my shoulders, but didn't say a word. Things had been going so well lately.

In an effort to expose my trickery, Mom supervised my tests for a week. My perfect streak was demolished by a 4+ the first morning. I was Diabetic again and a 'bad' boy for not taking better care of myself.

Steven's demands in the morning forced mom to give up her observations and I was doing my own unsupervised tests again by the end of the week. That week had taught me a valuable lesson; that too much of a good thing was 'bad'. I quickly revised my experiments so mom's suspicions wouldn't be aroused. I figured if I mixed things up a bit, a 3+ here, a 2+ there amongst mostly Trace and Negative results, my mom was kept happy and suspicion free. This false recording worked great, for almost three months. Then mom took me to a real lab and a nurse took several syringes full of blood for testing. That wasn't too bad but then a couple of days later I was taken to my first Doctor's visit outside of Sick Kids. That's when my clever façade fell apart.

Old Doc Weber lifted me up onto the examination table in his office and asked me if I'd brought my logbook. My Mom pulled it out of her purse and handed it to him saying," David's tests have been much better lately." There was pride in her voice, but I puffed up my chest.

The Doctor looked over every page of my log book. Then he opened my medical file. It was thick for a four year old. By this age I'd already put a railway spike through one foot and been bitten in the face by my own dog, requiring seventeen stiches and almost costing me an eye. He pulled out a sheet of paper. He examined it for a moment, scratched his balding head and looked through my log again.

I got the feeling something bad was going to happen. But he said, "The test results in your log are much better than I'd expected." I brightened right up at those words, having obviously fooled him too. Then he said, "Can you explain why they are so different from the Lab's test results. The Lab results were embarrassingly higher than the ones I'd so proudly and precisely colored into my log.

I blushed and shrugged my shoulders, unable to come up with a plausible explanation for the difference while under the glaring gaze of my mom. "You're not fooling anyone but yourself," she said in front of the Doctor. I was afraid the blood rushing to my head would cause it to explode, I was so embarrassed.

Doc Weber shook his head and said to my mom, "I think he needs to be told." My mom nodded and hung her head. "David, Diabetes can lead to blindness, amputation and death if you don't take better care of it. You have to do your tests properly, so I'll know how to help you. We're a team, you and I."

In the car on the way home I asked my mom what blindness and amputation were. Tears rolled down her cheeks as she explained. "Put your hands over your eyes, that's what blindness is, you can't see anything ever again. Amputation is when they have to cut off your leg." I don't remember saying much the rest of the ride home and went straight out to play road hockey with my newest best friend Craig.

When my Dad got home that night and heard about my Doctor visit he said, "You're not hurting anyone but yourself." My parents used catchy phrases and words of wisdom like that all the time. Between the two of them and the Doctor I got the message, "I wasn't hurting any fool but myself."

Now, after more than 50 years of regular daily testing, I live by two simple rules regarding the results. When my sugars are high, I take a needle, drink water and go for a walk. When they're low, I take a break, eat and drink.

Highs and lows will come and go. Deal with them the best you can. Live to stay healthy until the cure is found and available. That's what's important. That's the test.

Chapter 2
Sweet Tooth

I was once Dr. Mallory Banting. My grandfather was the illegitimate son of Sir Fredrick Banting. He discovered Insulin in 1921 while searching for a cure for Diabetes Mellitus. Insulin was a breakthrough treatment for Diabetes to be sure, but not its cure. He received the 1923 Nobel Prize for Medicine, then for no apparent reason abandoned his research into a cure. He died in a plane crash on his way to England to witness the birth of his son, my grandfather.

Throughout my life I have often wondered why he didn't finish the job? Did fame & notoriety get in his way? Was he seduced by more leisurely pursuits once he had wealth? Or was he simply satisfied with his contribution to the world? Maybe he just wanted to leave a mystery or two for the next generation to solve?

Whatever his reason, research into a cure for Diabetes ground to a halt for almost fifty years. Except in our family. His failure to find the cure has embarrassed as well as driven our family for four generations.

When my grandfather was old enough, my great grandmother encouraged him to become a great Doctor, like his father. All his life she spurred him on to complete Sir Banting's work and find the cure for Diabetes. "It's a matter of family honor," she told him time and time again.

Alas, my grandfather inherited none of his father's brilliance. Yet he did exceed Sir Banting's determination and spent his entire life in dogged pursuit of the cure. He spent little time with his wife and two boys, except to school them in what he'd learned. When my grandfather passed on, my father and uncle carried on his research. My father raised my older brother, twin sister and I to follow in the family business of searching for the cure, whether we liked it or not. Not, in my case.

After four generations of research, guess who gets the heavy responsibility of actually producing results. That great weight has landed squarely onto the narrow shoulders of my older brother, Dr. L.J. Banting, my evil twin sister Dr. Valerie Banting, and me. One of us had to cough up a cure, any cure, before some other scientist discovered one.

To better the odds of success, and steer clear of each other, we've each chosen a different field of research. L.J., a poorly controlled type 2 Diabetic himself, focused on the bio-mechanical cure. He is working on a project to develop a tiny mechanical Pancreas for surgical implantation.

Valerie preferred the surgical implantation of donor pancreas cells, protected from immune system response by a polymer coating.

According to their annoying, taunting texts, they're both really close to a cure.

Personally, I can't stand the sight of blood, so I chose the newest field of research, genetic reengineering. I'm creating a virus that will reprogram a Diabetic's genetic code so their immune system tolerates Insulin producing Beta cells, while at the same time triggering the regeneration of Beta cells in the Pancreas. Simply put, Diabetics catch a cold and get cured. My cure might even be contagious.

I'd never really given the research my all until three years ago when I was diagnosed with Type 1 Diabetes. Since that day I've dedicated my life to discovering its cure. Not for any misplaced sense of family honor, like the rest of my family. Not for good old, Sir Banting. Nope, I'm doing it for my own selfish reasons: self-preservation, fame, fortune, and a Nobel Prize.

Recently I've had several fantastic and unexpected breakthroughs. Yet, day after agonizing day, I've been denied the final breakthrough. It's frustrating me to the point of madness. I'm so close. I can almost see it sitting there at the dark, blurry edge of my mind. All I need is a spark of inspiration to illuminate it.

Lately, every genetic recombination experiment I've conducted has failed. I'm sacrificing every waking moment to solving this puzzle. I've stopped returning texts, e-mails, phone calls, and started ignoring visitors completely. I've even taken to sleeping at the Lab, obsessing over the problem late into the night.

After a couple of weeks of not eating right, or taking care of my Diabetes, my health began to suffer. Low blood sugar reactions stopped me dead in my tracks, demanding my full attention and eating up valuable time. My high sugars made it impossible to think clearly or control my emotions.

I began to botch simple experiments. Frustration and high sugars led to more and more frequent violent outbursts. The last time I smashed up the lab equipment pretty good. My boss was going to be furious.

I needed a break. Time to get back onto a routine, bring my sugars under control, and clear my head. I locked up my research, texted my boss that I was taking a sabbatical, and went camping in Algonquin Park. Fresh air and exercise have always made me feel better.

I checked the provincial weather forecasts for the next week. It had been a dry summer with no rain in the forecast. So I stuffed my backpack, hopped the first train north and caught a ride to the Park from a nice elderly couple I met at the Tim Horton's on highway 60.

They were going to their cottage, a couple of kilometers from the West gate. When they turned off the highway they let me out. I didn't feel like hiking the ten kms. to the Park office, just to register. Not when the Park border was right across the highway from where I was standing. I smiled my rebel smile, slung my backpack over my shoulder, ran across the highway and vanished between the trees. Thus began a hike that would change my life and that of every Diabetic in the world, forever.

* * * * *

On the sixth evening, deep in the park, according to my compass, I pitched camp high atop a grey granite bluff. I finished the operation just in time to observe another magnificent sunset. The dying sun lit up the sky, splashing the wispy clouds with a million dramatic shades of red.

"Red sky at night a scientist's delight," I improvised whimsically. In response, the wispy clouds turned a darker red, taking on the appearance of bloody claw marks scratched across the sky. I wanted to look away, hating the sight of blood, but at that exact moment, the breakthrough I'd been searching for exploded upon my mind. I sat bolt upright, staring at the horrific claw marks, but not seeing them. I had the answer.

I could hardly believe it. It couldn't be, not that simple. I went over it several times in my mind, until there could be no doubt about it. I'd done it!

I'd discovered the Cure for Diabetes.

Whipping out my cell phone and switching it on, praying for enough battery life to make the most important call of my life, maybe the most important call in all of human history. A terminal disease was about to be wiped off the face of the planet, thanks to me.

I waited an agonizing 10 seconds for it to power up and search for a signal. My eyes never leaving the tiny screen. I was desperate to tell the world of my discovery.

'NO SIGNAL' popped up on the screen.

"Shit. Shit, shit, shit," I fumed, holding my phone higher, then waving it in every direction, desperate to find a signal. Nothing. I gave up and shut it off before the battery wore out.

I was alone in the middle of nowhere on the greatest night of my life. I had to satisfy the primal need to express my triumph over Diabetes, over my brother and sister and every failed generation before me.

Leaping to my feet, I took a deep breath, put cupped hands to either side of my mouth, leaned back and gave a long mighty victory howl. The echo bounced between the surrounding hillsides, raising a chorus of animal cries, calls and howls in response.

Joyful tears filled my eyes and flowed freely down my cheeks, soaking my week old beard.

"I'm gonna be cured." I repeated aloud at least a dozen times. Then I started thinking about the material wealth my discovery would bring.

"I'm gonna be filthy rich & rock star famous the minute I get back to civilization. Nobel Prize for Medicine, come to poppa."

I was sorely tempted to try hiking out of the Park in the dark, but thought better of it. I was at least three days hike from the Park entrance. Instead, I busied myself making a cooking fire and pulling up a big sitting log. Then I pulled out the tan, leather bound, notebook L.J. had given me for my last birthday. I sat there a moment and excitedly scribbled the Cure's formula into it. I couldn't risk putting it in my smart phone, too much cyber crime and I wanted all the credit. As soon as I got back I was going straight to the patent office to register my cure. Then let the celebrations begin.

"Guess it wouldn't hurt to clean up a bit," I said rubbing my bristly jaw. It'd help pass the time, so I washed up, shaved and combed my hair, while visions of my brilliant new life danced before my mind's eye.

All fresh and clean, I sat on the log by the fire and rummaged through my backpack. Hunger was poking me in the stomach. I pulled out my small black bottomed copper pot and set it on on one of the flat rocks that ringed the fire, then took stock of my food. Including the wild vegetables and mushrooms collected along the trail and the box of biscuit mix, I had enough for my celebratory supper…Vegetarian Chili and biscuits, cooked over an open fire. Third time this week, and to tell you the truth, I was getting pretty sick of it.

I deserved to dine with Royalty for what I'd done tonight damn it! But all the rewards would have to wait thanks to the lack of microwave towers in this God forsaken forest. I took a deep breath to calm myself. No sense getting all worked up, gotta watch my blood pressure, don't want to have a stroke. I took a second deep breath. For now, a meager meal and planning my brilliant future would have to suffice.

My sugars were 5.5 when I tested, perfect. I chose not to take a needle, but knew I'd better eat soon or risk a reaction and end up dining on Dextrose (sugar tablets). I'd packed lots in case of emergency. Taking out the tube I'd almost emptied earlier in the day, due to a couple of reactions, I shook out the last two tablets into my mouth, chewed and swallowed. That ought to keep my sugars level until I ate. Pitching the empty tube into the fire, I turned around to toss my tester into my backpack.

I heard the fire crackle and settle. Then the ever-present chirping of crickets faded into an eerie silence. I stopped what I was doing to listen. Nearby bird-calls ceased. A gentle breeze carried a damp chill through camp making the short hairs on the back of my neck stand at attention. There was a faint earthy odor in the night air and I sensed a presence.

My first thought was, "You're early tonight." For the past few evenings, shortly after sunset, my campsite had been frequented by several freeloading squirrels, and a ravenous raccoon. I'd taken to tossing them my dinner scraps while sitting by the campfire. On the second night, I'd started whispering to them of my search for the cure while they ate. Boy, did I have news for them tonight.

I turned around slowly, so as not to scare them away. But instead of a hungry little animal, I saw a beautiful native woman slip from the blackness of the forest, silent as a shadow. She just stood there at the edge of the firelight, staring at me.

"Oh man. Fate is truly smiling on me tonight!" I thought, and gave her a great big smile while raising my hand in silent greeting. She didn't respond at first. Her head just turned slightly, as if she'd heard a faint distant sound, but her eyes never left mine. She seemed to be sizing me up.

I must have met with her approval. She moistened her luscious lips with the tip of her tongue and said, "Hi, I'm Giinibide." She had a sexy, playful voice. "Call me Giini," she added with a wave of her hand. "I saw your fire from my camp over there." She waved a hand off to her right. "Ummmm, something sure smells good, mind if I stay for a bite?"

I stood and gestured towards the space on the log next to me. "Please do, I can't imagine a more perfect dinner companion. I'm Mallory, Mallory Banting and I've just discovered the cure for Diabetes."

Giini raised a respectful eyebrow and nodded once, smiling broadly. "Congratulations, you must be pumped," she said.

It was my turn to raise an eyebrow. Had she read my mind? Or did we have the same thing on our minds? "Pumped is a good word," I replied cooly.

I took silent pleasure in watching her feline gracefulness as she glided around the fire and sat down beside me without making a sound.

She was exquisite looking. Shiny, raven black hair, braided down her back, high cheekbones and hypnotic dark green, almost black eyes. Her skin was flawless, her teeth straight and white.

"Care to share," I said nodding towards the simmering pot of chili.

"No thanks, I grabbed a bite at sunset, but I'm up for dessert," she purred. I knew we were talking about the same thing when she licked her smiling lips and gave me an alluring wink.

We gazed into each others' eyes and exchanged some casual small talk heavily laced with sexual innuendo. She told me her name was Ojibway for 'sharp tooth', and bit at me playfully. "Strange name" I thought, but didn't really give a crap. Her name could have meant 'no tooth' and I'd have found her just as arousing. There was something about her I found totally irresistible.

Experience told me to eat something before we got busy, but I was more horny than hungry at this point. Besides it'd spoil the mood and I really wanted to celebrate with her, damn it!

As if reading my mind, Giini tenderly took my hand, stood and led me to my tent. She pulled back the door flap and guided me inside.

I'd never been with such a sexual wildcat before. Squirming and wriggling beneath me. Scratching then clawing my back, grabbing hold and rolling me onto my back. Once on top she started licking and nibbling me here, there and *everywhere*. I quickly learned why she'd been named sharp tooth. Her teeth were like tiny razors, actually nicking my skin several times. I couldn't see if she'd drawn blood, but it sure felt like it.

I didn't complain though, simply because each time she pained me, she quickly pleasured me to the point that all I could do was moan in ecstasy.

She'd nuzzled and nibbled her way from my nipples to my neck when without warning she bit down hard. I mean break the skin hard. Christ it hurt! I swear she took a chunk out of me. Something wet started trickling down my neck.

"Oh no, blood," I thought. Thank god I couldn't see it or I'd pass right out. As it was, I felt woozy. Then I heard the distinct sound of sucking next to my left ear. "Oh God, this crazy bitch is sucking the blood from my wound?! What'd she think she was, a fucking Vampire?"

The thought of all the diseases she could be transmitting was enough to make me fight desperately to get free of her. Giini just latched on tighter. Man she was strong. Horrific as the situation was, it gave me an erection like an iron rod. Giini went wild, moaning and groaning, but staying glued to my throat. We were really going at it, when my blood sugars crashed. I started sweating, but felt cold.

Giini abruptly stopped gyrating. She pulled her teeth from my throat with a wet sucking sound and sat back. I slowly raised my hand and applied weak pressure to the vicious wound in my throat. I looked up at Giini, searching her face for the reason behind this attack, but she was unconcerned with me.

She was too busy swishing my blood around in her mouth. It gave her the appearance of a discriminating wine connoisseur. All at once she turned her head and spat it out in disgust.

"You're a damned Diabetic!?" she screamed at me, exposing long blood soaked fangs.

"You're a damned Vampire!?" I screamed back in nauseous terrified disbelief.

I struggled furiously to disengage myself from her, but Giini was having none of it. She thumped a remarkably heavy clawed hand onto my chest, pinning me in place. Weak from loss of blood and plummeting blood sugars, I was at her mercy, and she knew it.

"Well this changes everything," she started. "Guess I'll have to kill you now, before you turn. What a shame, I really liked you, but you gotta die," she sounded truly sorry. Helplessly, I watched as she slowly, almost reluctantly, raised her right clawed hand to strike me dead. I closed my eyes.

But instead of feeling pain, I heard something tear through my tent wall. I opened my eyes. A silver dagger tip was paused just above my left eye. It was so close I could see that some bizarre ancient runes were etched into it. The blade held Giini's attention too. It only hesitated for a second, then it zipped away towards my feet, cleanly slicing my tent wall in half.

"Oh thank God we're being robbed," I thought. Given the current situation, I'd rather be robbed at knife point than killed by a disappointed Vampire.

Two beefy hands burst through the gash and grabbed Giini by her hair. She screamed as she was yanked off me and out of the tent. Sounds of a violent struggle erupted close by, quickly growing fainter as the fighting moved off.

I lay there, too weak to move. My heart pounding heavily in my chest. I lay there, listening as each beat grew weaker, fainter. Boom boom, Boom boom...Boom, boom...boom, boom...boom...boom....

In the end my heart quivered once and stopped. I was dead, and thoroughly disappointed. How did the greatest night of my life turn into this fatal surreal nightmare.

A relaxing calm swept over me like a warm tropical breeze. I expected a bright light to appear and take me away, or maybe a velvety blackness smothering my existence, or even a transition to a higher plane of existence, something. But nothing happened. I just lay there, dead calm.

Then the faintest pins and needles sensation started in the pit of my stomach, spreading like wild fire consuming my body, leaving me cold and numb.

This was nothing like what I thought being dead would feel like. This felt like my lowest blood sugar reaction ever. I loathed this feeling.

To make matters worse, the numbness in my stomach was growing into an emptiness. I was so empty it hurt.

It took all my strength, but I managed to roll out of my tent through the gash in the tent wall. Once outside I forced myself to stand, bloody, naked and starving. Now what? Grunting and loud panting spun me around.

Silhouetted by the campfire's flickering light were the forms of two struggling women. I instantly recognized Giini's supple naked body nearest the fire. She was propping herself up with her right arm, supporting her weight and that of her adversary, a fair haired, muscular woman nearly twice Giini's size. She was trying to drive the tent-slicing dagger into Giini's chest using both hands.

Giini had a poor left-handed grip on the woman's right wrist, which only slowed the blade's steady advance. She was in trouble.

The big woman kept deftly shifting her weight, to counter Giini's struggling and gain the advantage. They were both panting and dripping sweat from the effort. Then it struck me, this wasn't a robbery as I'd first suspected. I was witnessing a fight to the death.

With a powerful grunt, the big woman shifted her weight. Giini's supporting arm collapsed beneath them. It was pinned badly behind her back, forcing an angry, desperate, painful scream past her clenched teeth.

The big woman seized the moment, pushing the blade an inch closer. It grazed Giini's breast. The struggle was nearly over. Giini pushed back with all her strength, but the blade only moved a fraction of an inch from her bosom.

"I thought you'd be stronger," taunted the blonde woman.

"Who are you?" panted Giini.

Through clenched yellow teeth, the big woman snarled, "Jane White..." Twisting the dagger, further weakening Giini's grip on it, she added "...Vampire Hunter." Giini bared her fangs and hissed at her.

"You got my partner at dusk," spat Jane, moving her face closer to Giini's, she lowered her voice menacingly, "Missed me though." Then her voice grew louder, "But I'm not gonna miss you... Vampire!" She reared her head and shoulders back, then drove the dagger down with all her strength.

The tip of the dagger cut into Giini's left breast, red flame and sparks shot out of the wound. She let out an inhuman roar of excruciating pain that sent a shiver up my spine.

Giini began writhing and twitching in such desperate agony, I couldn't help feeling sorry for her. If I was going to do something to help, it was now or never.

But, what to do? Who to help? Then the breeze shifted direction and the answer hit me right between the eyes, literally. I was overwhelmed by the smell of toasted marshmallows, honey, chocolate and vanilla ice cream. It was a sickly sweet odor that saturated the air and filled my every breath. I was drawn to it like a moth to a flame.

I lifted my nose, sniffing the night air. No doubt about it, the smell came from Jane. The Vampire Hunter's rapid, heavy breathing was creating a fog of irresistible sweetness, carried to me on the night breeze. It was so thick and strong I could almost see it.

My breathing became rapid & shallow, a raw animalistic power surged through my veins. Every muscle, nerve and fiber of my being was electrified. I felt stronger and hungrier than I'd ever felt before. I crouched low, then launched myself at the big woman, covering the 10 meters between us in a single bound.

Problem was, I'd propelled myself too high and fast, I was going to overshoot my target. Then, just for a moment, time slowed. As my naked form shot by overhead, Jane turned and looked up. Her eyes widened in horror. I twisted around in midair like some demonic acrobat, reaching down and grabbing her by the shoulders, tearing her off Giini. Then time returned to it's normal speed.

I landed with the perfect footing and plenty of momentum to swing the big woman over my head in a huge arc and slam her to the ground, flat on her back. She went limp and the dagger slipped from her hand.

I did a one handed cartwheel and landed in a sitting position atop her belly. Her body pulsed beneath my naked buttocks. This close, I was dizzy with the smell of her sugary blood. I craved it. That realization gave me pause. What had happened to my revulsion, nausea, and fainting at the sight of blood? Here I was happily about to kill a woman in order to drink her blood. I smiled at the irony.

Jane regained consciousness at that point, shaking her head and squinting up curiously at my smiling, unfamiliar face. Her eyes quickly widened, as did mine, when my fangs grew out for the first time. A strange, but not unpleasant sensation.

I ran a curious tongue over my enlarged canines while my dinner thrashed about frantically trying to escape. She swept her hand across the ground trying to locate her dagger.

"Stop playing with your food and eat!" Giini interrupted, "We need to talk."

As a Doctor, I'd sworn an oath to do no harm, but my ravenous hunger rapidly devoured my ethics & morality, finally consuming my very soul. I became its unwilling slave, powerless to resist.

Jane found her dagger, but before she could use it against me, I struck, quick like a snake, sinking my fangs deep into her throbbing carotid artery.

Her flesh was warm and had the consistency of a juicy tomato, but tasted sweeter than honey. My fangs tore her throat open a bit more and her sweet, hot blood gushed down my throat. As I fed, her heartbeat slowed and weakened until I had to suck out the last satisfying drops. Then to my surprise, I irreverently tossed aside her dry withered husk.

Her remains hit the ground with a hollow thud, and in that instant the last vestige of my humanity evaporated and I turned. One moment Human, the next, Vampire, a being who must kill and drink blood to live, and would live forever.

"I really aughta kill you," said Giini, getting to her feet and popping her dislocated shoulder back into the socket with a loud crunch.

"I had no idea you were a Diabetic when I bit you, sorry." She sounded almost regretful.

"Is that a problem?" I asked, wiping blood from the corners of my mouth with the back of my hand. If she wanted another fight, I was ready this time.

"Problem? humm, in a way. Vampires despise Diabetics, we call them 'Sweets'. Hard to find one that isn't too sweet & dry, or too wet and salty," she said, crinkling her eyes shut, sticking her tongue out between her full lips, hunching her shoulders and trembling to show her revulsion, then adding "Yuck."

"Hey!" I exclaimed, mildly offended. I didn't give a bat's ass if Vampires liked the taste of my blood or not, but, for some uncharacteristic reason, I did care that Giini hated it.

"Awww, don't be so sensitive lover. You tasted amazing, till your sugars dropped. Besides, it's not just about taste. Feeding on a Sweet's thick sugary blood slows our reflexes. Feeding on Sweets with low blood sugars, like yours were, weakens and confuses us. Either way, we become vulnerable to Hunters, as you just witnessed," she explained as I watched her wounded breast heal before my eyes. Incredible.

Giini turned and glided over to the fire, pausing just long enough to pull my sleeping bag from my ruined tent. She sat down cross legged on the ground in front of the fire and wrapped the sleeping bag around her shoulders. Then, turning her head, she looked at me, patting the earth beside her, "Come on over, I won't bite...again, unless you want me to," she teased, flashing a seductive smile.

I smiled back, relieved, then shivered. A chill had crept into the dry night air. Still naked, I gathered some wood for the fire, then sat down beside my Vampire tutor. She draped the sleeping bag over my shoulders as I sat. Giini's gorgeous body glistened in the firelight, but her eyes reflected the fire, becoming two flickering flames as she spoke of my new life.

"No Vampire has ever turned a Diabetic on purpose. It's cruel, and although you may have heard otherwise, we are not without compassion." Giini turned and stared into the fire in silence for a moment, pondering our predicament, I assumed.

"Okay listen, you saved my life, so I'm not going to take yours," she said. Then her eyebrows leapt up as if she'd just had a revelation. Slapping my knee lightly, and nodding her head, she added, "In fact, I'm gonna teach you the three basic rules we Vampires live by."

"First, and most important: *Stay in your Range.* We Vampires are extremely territorial. In an age long forgotten, there were so many Vampires in the world, food became scarce," she began.

"What? You mean to tell me Humans were an endangered species," I asked, shocked at the revelation.

"Yup. Vampires, and their bloodlines, fought each other over the remaining food. Their battles swept over the planet like a plague for centuries.

The final Vampire battle over the world's remaining food supply occurred early in the 13th century. Human history records it as the Bubonic plague, *the Black Death.* A full third of Europe's Human population was wiped out, but more importantly, hundreds of Vampire bloodlines were either decimated, or killed off completely.

After that battle only the original Vampires remained, one from each branch of the human race. They proclaimed themselves 'Royal' Vampires and convened a Royal Court. The goal of the court was to divide the world into Hunting 'Ranges', one Range for each Royal Vampire. They figured that was the only way to keep the peace and still have enough food for each Vampire's feeding needs.

I hear there were thousands of Ranges at first. About that time the Human race discovered the existence of Vampires and what a horrific threat they were. We hunters quickly became the hunted as the first Vampire Hunters appeared."

This was amazing to me, that an entire race of flesh eaters had co-evolved with Humans since the dawn of our species. I sat in silent amazement as Giini continued.

"In the beginning, Hunters just murdered any feeding Vampire they stumbled across. Their methods were clumsy and crude. But every once in a while they got lucky and unwittingly murdered a Royal, wiping out every last Vampire in their bloodline.

Upon a Royal's death, their Range was either conquered by a neighboring Vampire, divided amongst neighboring Vampires, or became a Free Range where any registered Vampire can hunt.

Free Ranges are the best, just buy a tag and you can kill your quota. Algonquin Park is part of a Free Range, that's why I'm here.

Back on my Royal's Range, all the food is processed and raised in tall buildings. It's so commercialized. She made it sound like shopping in a grocery store. "If there's no challenge in a hunt, no fight in the prey, there's no taste in the meat. It's so boring, I hate it," she confided in a tense whisper as if we might be overheard.

"Why not just hunt somewhere else, like another Range," I asked.

"No way, that's considered poaching. If I got caught, they'd stake me out for the morning sun. Tssss boom."

"So all that Vampire lore I've heard about growing up, it's all true?" Another frosty shiver raced up my spine.

Yeah, kinda spooky eh?" she agreed. "But don't worry Sweety, it'll be different for you. You'll only be eating Diabetics, and normal Vampires don't, so you won't be cutting into their food supply. You can hunt where you like if you're careful who you eat. If I were you, I'd stick to hunting Vampire Hunters, you won't offend any Vampires by eating them."

"So, what? I'm a damned Vampire on a diet!" I cursed fate's cruel irony. Giini just laughed. "Well, look at it this way, now you can eat all the Sweets you like." I shot her a sarcastic half grin.

"Anyway," said Giini, "Second rule: *Eat light*. Killing too many, or too often, will attract Vampire Hunters. They're Diabetics like you, recruited from support groups, trained to hunt us down and kill us." She kicked Jane's sack of bones carcass. "Kind of ominous your first meal was a Hunter, don't you think?" she added.

"But if you're going to feed on Hunters you better be on your game. They are numerous, organized and relentless." She cocked her head towards Jane's remains, "That one and her partner have been after me for three years. Once they catch you, they'll torture you for the whereabouts of our Royal, then kill you," She turned to me and caught me peeking under the sleeping bag at her naked body. Even splattered with sweat and dirt as it was, her body was exquisite and desirable.

"Pay attention, this is important," she chastised and I reluctantly drew my eyes back to her face and listened.

"Third rule: *Less is More*. Vampires can't reproduce like Humans, so we turn Humans into Vampires. But we are very selective as to who we turn. The Royal at the head of each bloodline dictates the criteria. We Vampires must keep our population stable. Uncontrolled increases in Vampire numbers would lead us back to starvation and war.

The fewer Diabetic Vampires you create, the more food you'll have. Each Vampire you create extends our Royal's bloodline and ties their very existence to his. It helps to think of those you turn as your children, you know, mouths to feed and all that. You're going to live a very long time if you're careful, eat right and protect our Royal."

"How ironic," I thought. "I'd said the exact same thing to countless Diabetic patients, everything except the 'protect our Royal' part."

Well if what Giini was saying was true, then I needed a lot more information if I was going to survive.

"Yeah, yeah, protect our Royal, but more importantly how often do Vampires feed? Do I still have to test my blood and take needles? Now that I'm one of the undead, can a low blood sugar reaction still kill me?" I asked concerned and hopeful. Maybe I could find a way back to my life with the brilliant future.

"I don't know about that stuff, I guess you'll just have to find out for yourself," said Giini.

"Will my Cure for Diabetes work on me now?"

Giini answered as best she could, obviously out of her depth, "As far as I know, you can't be cured of Diabetes, or any other diseases for that matter. If you have a disease when you turn, you're stuck with it. Come to think of it, a 'Cure for Diabetes' is now a threat to you. If you can't stop a Cure from being discovered, it'll destroy your food supply!"

A breeze carried smoke from the fire into my eyes making me wince and tear up. An electrified chill ran up my spine as I felt my family's torch fall from my hands.

I turned and looked Giini in the eyes. "Tonight, for the briefest of moments, I touched my place in history, I was the man who cured Diabetes. Savior to half a billion Diabetics worldwide. Now, according to you, instead of their savior I've become their bloodthirsty executioner and the anti-cure of Diabetes. I think I'm going to be sick." I turned to look into the fire, pulling the sleeping bag tighter around me. Giini put one arm around my shoulders and placed a hand on my knee, patting it softly. We sat in silence for a while.

Then a faint, familiar tingling started in the pit of my stomach. My sugars were dropping again.

Apparently I'd have to feed more than once a night. Instinctively I turned and grabbed a tube of liquid Dextrose from my nearby backpack. I needed sugar fast.

"Don't. Eat Sweets," blurted Giini cryptically when she saw what I was doing, but it was too late, I'd already swallowed the lifesaving liquid. I vomited immediately, spewing into the fire causing an explosion of sparks and thick smoke.

"I tried to warn you, Vampires can only feed on blood," said Giini turning aside while I wiped the spittle from my mouth. "Whadaya mean, I can't raise my blood sugars with anything but someone's sugary blood?" The thought of such a bloodthirsty existence turned my stomach in a couple of different directions.

As if that wasn't bad enough, the blood Hunger started clawing at my flipping stomach. I doubled over in pain. "Help me Giini, please," I pleaded. "I'll do anything." Giini smiled.

She stood up and taking my cold trembling hands, helped me to my feet. The sleeping bag fell to the ground and I gave an involuntary shiver.

"Okay, I'll help, but I'm only doing this cause you asked so nice," said Giini. "There's a campsite, due west, about 5 kms., mostly Diabetics. No food there for me, so I avoided them earlier. But now I think the Hunters we killed tonight, traveled into the Park with them, so while you're grabbing a bite, I'll check around for any more. If I find any you can have them. How does that sound?"

"Five K? I can't run nearly that far, with my sugars dropping," I advised her, hoping she had a closer, quicker, solution.

"Who said anything about running Sweety? Boy you have a lot to learn about being a Vampire," she teased. Giini made a high-pitched sound. Several large bats showed up a moment later, squeaking and flapping their leathery wings around our heads. In a remarkable display of speed, Giini snatched one out of the air and told me to do the same.

She taught me a magic spell then told me to bite the bat. "Vampires can take on the form of any mammal they bite", she said when I gave her a look of disgust. "You want food fast, bats can fly," she added.

So I closed my eyes, repeated the spell and chomped down on the hairy little snack. It squealed and struggled for a second, but before I could suck the bat dry a wave of electric heat swept over me.

In the blink of an eye . I was no longer on my feet, I was flapping my wings, hovering a meter in the air and echo-locating my surroundings. Very cool, I must admit, but there was no time to revel in the experience. Even as a bat I suffered the hunger pains. Giini the bat, squeaked at me and led the way as we flapped off towards the camp.

The spell only lasted a few minutes, just long enough for us to reach our destination. The instant our tiny, clawed feet touched the ground we changed back into human form, naked as when we'd left.

Giini put a hand on my shoulder and whispered in my ear. "Eat as few as you need to feel better, but no more. I'm gonna scout around, maybe grab a bite myself. I'll meet you back here in a half hour." I patted her hand twice to signal my agreement. She glided off between two tents.

I looked around wondering where to start. There were a dozen tents of all descriptions arranged in a loose circle around the campfire. There were no lights on inside any of them. The rock ringed campfire was little more than smoldering coals. Several empty bags of giant sized marshmallows leaned against the rocks.

Silly buggers must have been sitting around the fire, toasting marshmallows, laughing and eating one after another, til their sugars were so high they couldn't stop.

I caught the strong smell of sugar as the breeze changed direction. The sweetest smelling tent was across the camp. Steeling my will to the task, I leapt over the fire and silently entered. What I saw inside that tent made my skin crawl.

The alluring sweetness I'd detected was the breath and body odor of a Sumo sized, fat guy. He was lying on his back, half-naked, snoring and sweating. Gross!!

I didn't care how low my sugars got, or how badly the Hunger tore at me, I wasn't biting another man's neck. Heck, he hadn't even shaved. I fought down my homophobic nausea, turned and soundlessly staggered from the tent.

Time was running out. My fingertips started tingling, then one by one went numb. Swaying and weaving I made my way to the tent next door and entered.

Two plump young women were sleeping inside. Hunger lanced my belly, doubling me over. Then a madness possessed me and my fangs shot down. My clawed hands were spread like wings and with surgical perfection, I slashed both their throats open simultaneously. I'd cut deep enough to sever their vocal chords. Although their eyes opened wide in surprised horror, and their hands went to their severed throats, they made no sound, except burbling gasps as their lungs filled with blood.

Their blood started spurting everywhere, covering the tents walls and ceiling with hideous patterns. I closed my eyes, but opened my mouth and stuck out my tongue to catch the drops.

Normally, long before now, I'd have vomited and passed out, but I was possessed and forced to endure.

When the first drops of blood splashed over my taste buds it was an orgasmic experience. That's the only way I can describe it.

Then I swallowed. It felt like honey flowing down my throat. When it hit my stomach the starvation eased a bit. A second later power surged throughout my body and my mind was filled with one thought "MORE!"

Before I knew it I was at the first woman's throat sucking away like a hungry baby. I drained her in seconds flat. I paused as the hunger faded, my sugars rose and the power within grew immense. I felt practically superhuman.

I turned and glared at the second woman. She hadn't moved. Frozen in terror, helpless, defenseless and still spurting blood. I affixed myself to her wound without a struggle and for an instant I understood what Giini had meant by no fight, no flavor.

When I finished her off the madness evaporated. My mind was my own again and the Hunger had abated. My reaction was gone and the power coursing through me, oh man the power, I felt invincible. But before I could exit the blood soaked tent, a thought wormed its' way into my mind, "What would happen if I ate just one more?"

Crouched between the two corpses, I pondered a truly morbid experiment. How to determine the amount each feeding raised my blood sugars? I'd have to check my sugars before & after I fed. Plus check my victim's blood sugars before I drained them completely. It was a gruesome way to learn what to eat & how much, but it had to be done. First thing I needed was a glucometer, mine was back at my camp.

Quietly rummaging around the women's tent I found one glucometer. I'd use the first test as a starting point and see how much the next meal raised them.

I pricked my finger, but no blood appeared. Even after much squeezing I got no blood. Only after pricking myself several times in the same spot did I finally get a tiny drop of blood, barely large enough for test. The result was 8.5.

Now, normally I wouldn't eat anything if my sugars were this high, but I was curious. Besides, what harm could come from eating one or maybe two more Sweets. I was conducting an experiment, not planning a banquet. I waited fifteen minutes then tested again. 8.0. That meant my sugars were dropping 2 points every hour. I had to feed again tonight, that much was obvious to me.

I began my feeding experiment with the old lady I found asleep in the tent next door. A half eaten bag of marshmallows lay by her cot. I drained her of all but the necessary drop for the test. Her sugars were 20.1. "A real sweet old lady," I chuckled to myself.

I tested my sugars 11.5. That sweet old lady had only raised my sugars 3 points, almost nothing. I'd better try again, one last bite for the night, then I'd stop and go find Giini, maybe fool around some more before my sugars got too high and she couldn't stand the smell of me.

As I left the old lady's tent I caught a whiff of sweetness on the breeze. All thoughts of finding Giini turned to thoughts of finding the source of that sweetness.

After my third meal my sugars were 18.9, and I had a voracious hunger growing by the second. It's a well-documented medical fact that Diabetics with sugars over 15.5, develop an insatiable appetite. The more they eat, the higher their sugars go. The higher their sugars go, the more ravenous their hunger becomes. It's a vicious cycle made all the worse by Vampirism.

I thought about finding Giini, but every time I left one tent I'd catch a whiff of syrupy sweetness coming from another tent across the camp. I tried to resist, but the odor clouded my mind and I had to follow my nose.

When Giini found me I was finishing off my twelfth sweet meal... the disgusting fat guy I'd passed on earlier.

"What a pig!!" she scolded with a furrowed brow. At first I thought she was referring to my meal. Then I realized she was insulting me for how I was eating, not what.

Like a starving dog with a choice bone, my fangs never left the guy's bristly throat. I just stared back at her defiantly. I was ready to tear her apart if she tried to remove my meal before I'd finished. I was so full of power I could barely control it. Giini took a step towards me. I gave a low warning growl, then went back to my meal, sucking harder and faster.

She waved her hand at the campsite now littered with corpses. "This kinda carnage is what alerts Vampire Hunters to our whereabouts." She swore in Ojibway and stamped her foot. "What were you thinking?"

My feeding frenzy was a bit foggy to me. By the looks of things I'd been dragging Diabetics from their tents while still feeding on them, then carelessly discarding their spent corpses all over the camp. For some bizarre reason their corpses reminded me of fast food litter.

Giini snapped her fingers in front of my nose to regain my attention. My eyes locked onto her.

"We'll have to burn this whole mess tonight. It'll take a forest fire to explain all these corpses. We better hurry too, it'll be sunrise soon."

I grunted and finished off the fat guy, tossing his husk over my shoulder. I was still insanely hungry, but there wasn't anyone left.

Fighting the urge to bite Giini, I busied myself helping her set fires in the tinder dry forest, then quickly tested my sugars. They were 34.0. They'd never been so high before, but I wasn't worried.

I knew my sugars would drop without me having to take a needle. That was a plus, no more needles, but I had no idea when I'd have to eat again. What if they bottomed out during the day while I slept. It wasn't like I could get up and go out for a snack in the light if the legends about Vampires were true. Guess I'd have to "wait and see" like Giini had said earlier.

When the forest was ablaze behind us, we summoned bats and flew to Giini's 'Safe House', a cave deep in the rugged heart of the Park not far from my campsite. When I mentioned this fact to Giini she told me to go there and erase any trace of my having been there.

I raced over to my site, packed it up and brought it to Giini's cave. I got there just as the first rays of the morning sun colored the sky. I stood there admiring it at the cave's entrance until Giini grabbed my arm and hauled me deeper into the blackness of her cave. It took a second for my eyes to adjust, but then I saw just fine. Surprisingly well in fact.

"Don't be so reckless," said Giini over her shoulder. Her hand slipped down my arm. "Daylight will kill you, quick as a wink," she warned, taking my hand. The cave extended some hundred feet or so into the rock, twisting and turning several times, but the dry rock floor always sloped downward.

We walked in silence for a spell, hand in hand, then the ceiling lifted away and we stepped into a vast cavern.

"You can sleep here today, with me, but you can't stay," she said apologetically. "You know I like you, way more than I should, but if you can't learn to control your sweet tooth you'll attract Hunters like flies to honey," she cautioned. "Bad for you is bad for us. Vampires won't tolerate you on their Range for long if Hunters are tracking you there."

I nodded my understanding. She showed me over to a raised section of smooth rock about the size of two king sized beds. I unslung my backpack, letting it drop to the floor.

We climbed onto the rock bed and made small talk for a couple of minutes, but Giini was having trouble keeping her eyes open. Finally she yawned, smiled and kissed me. Then she rolled onto her back, folded her arms over her chest and went straight to sleep without another word.

Lay there considering all that Giini had told me, and warned me about, I came up with a plan of action.

I'd hunt where Sweets were most plentiful...Diabetes support groups. I'd visit every last one, in every town and city of the world. No Diabetic with high sugars could hide, not even the Vampire Hunters. I'd hunt and kill them in each Range I travelled through. That ought to ingratiate me with the local Vampires.

I tested my sugars one last time before sleep. They were 26.1. Changing into a bat sure burned up a lot of sugar. I calculated the rate of decline and figured I had almost 14 hours before they'd fall to levels demanding I feed again. Well after sunset.

With my sugars at a safe level, a bed to rest upon, and a plan to follow, I let sleep take me. I was naked, on my back, with my arms folded across my chest...right next to a Vampire. I slept like a baby.

We both awoke at sunset, sitting up at the same time like an alarm had gone off. I felt surprisingly well rested, energized in fact but the air was chilly. I rolled off the warm rock bed and started to make a fire. Gini went off to pee.

There was a pile of small sticks stacked against the back wall.

I tore pages from my journal, the ones with the formula for the Cure, crumpling them into balls and placing them amongst the sticks. As I struck the match to light the pages, a sense of great loss struck me. Maybe I should hang onto these pages, they were the only proof of what I'd accomplished. But another chill ran up my spine, making me shiver, so I put the flame to the pages to keep warm. "No profit in a cure anyway," I whispered under my breath and sighed.

After warming up a bit, I tested my sugars. They were 7.0. I hoped that was acceptable to her, if I really had to leave, I wanted Giini one last time. Chances were we'd never see each other again after tonight.

When Giini returned she told me I smelled good, in a playful voice. We made love Vampire style, sucking each other's blood as we did it. (Best sex ever!). Afterwards we lay there naked, just talking for a while. We'd have laid there all night except our hunger for Blood soon replaced our hunger for each other.

We crawled up from the depths of the cave and breathed in the cool night air. It stank of smoke and ash. Having no more use for it I placed my journal atop a rock at the mouth of the cave. Standing there watching the final color drain from the sky Giini turned and gave me a long passionate kiss. During that kiss, I realized that despite her ending my life, career, and dreams with a single bite, I'd miss her.

Our lips parted and she smiled at me. "See ya round, Sweet Tooth." As she spoke, she stepped away from me and glided back into the black of the surrounding forest. I watched her until she completely disappeared, just the reverse of how she'd first appeared to me.

"No sense standing here burning sugars," I said aloud. I held a wetted finger in the air. The wind abruptly changed and blew to the south, towards Toronto. "Hmmm, lots of Diabetics there," I mused. I summoned a bat and as I held out its wings about to chant the spell I remembered that my brother lived in Toronto, and he was a type 2 Diabetic. Maybe I'd stop in and see how his research was going, grab a bite, chew the fat. After all, he was such a sweet guy.

Chapter 3
Sick Kids Stay

1967 was an eventful year: Canada celebrated its 100th birthday. Expo 67 opened in Montreal. Disney released 'Jungle Book'. The Monkees won an Emmy. Mohammed Ali won the World Heavyweight title. Evil Knievel jumped sixteen cars on a motorcycle. Toronto Maple Leafs beat the Montreal Canadians for the Stanley Cup. US and USSR conducted provocative monthly underground nuclear tests. DNA was created in a test tube. The 1st human heart transplant was performed in South Africa and I was held captive in a Canadian hospital for six torturous weeks.

November of that year I was captured by sweet talking Nurses at The Hospital for Sick Children in Toronto. Commonly referred to as 'Sick Kids'.

A couple of days earlier I'd gone outside with wet hair after swimming lessons, despite my Mother's repeated warnings not to. All the kids were doing it, combing their wet hair flat against their scalps. We looked like poster children for hair gel. Outside in the cold autumn air my hair quickly froze into a helmet, I caught cold as soon as it thawed when I got home.

My cold worsened by the hour until I could barely draw breath. When I did manage to snatch a breath it brought on a wet racking coughing fit. My parents rushed me to Sick Kid's despite my not wanting to go, but I was too weak to argue.

Five years earlier they'd taken me to Sick Kids where I'd been examined and diagnosed with Diabetes. This time I was examined and diagnosed with double pneumonia. The two don't mix well. I was admitted immediately.

In the Emergency room, a curtain was drawn around me & a bed. I got undressed and put on a standard issue powder blue hospital gown. Yes, the kind that ties in back, but doesn't close in back, exposing your bum to everyone. I piled my clothes at the foot of the bed. The effort undressing and dressing exhausted me, so I hopped up and lay down on the examining room bed.

I swear, no sooner had I closed my eyes, than a Nurse pulled back the curtain, gathered up my clothes and gave them to my waiting parents. The realization I wasn't going home tonight forced its way into my mind.

A second Nurse entered and helped lift me from the examining bed onto a gurney. The two nurses covered me in warm blankets, then raised & locked the gurney's silver side rails in place. An oxygen mask was placed over my nose & mouth, its clear flexible tube connected to the silver oxygen cylinder under my gurney.

One of the Nurses grabbed the metal clip board with my medical chart and laid it across my legs. It was heavy.

"Okay here we go" said the Nurse kicking off the bed's wheel brakes. She rolled me & the bed out of the examining room and down the hall. Exhausted & helpless, I lay there looking up as the fluorescent ceiling lights flicked by on our way to the elevator. I wasn't scared, just anxious. I didn't know where I'd be sleeping tonight, in a room or in the hall. I'd been trapped and held captive for short periods in several hospitals before. Whenever a room wasn't available, I'd slept on a gurney in the hall.

We waited for the first elevator to arrive in a vestibule with four elevator doors, two on our right, two on our left. There were two triangular lights above each set of elevator doors. Together they looked like two halves of a diamond to me.

When the elevator arrived, the triangle pointing up turned green quickly followed by a "Bing" sound.

The elevator's stainless steel double doors slid open. I was wheeled inside by one nurse while the other said, "Good night, I hope you're better soon," then she headed back towards the Emergency room.

My gurney rumbling horribly as its wheels crossed the gap between floor and elevator car. I reflexively clutched at the side rails to steady myself.

Inside the elevator car a mellow instrumental version of a popular song was playing. The sliding doors closed and for a second nothing happened. Suddenly with a jolt the elevator, and a noisy air conditioner, started up.

My Mom held my hand lovingly from one side of the gurney while my Dad gave my shoulder a reassuring squeeze from the other. The Nurse examined my chart. We rode straight up to my floor without stopping.

There was a muffled "Bing!" when we reached our floor. The air conditioner squeaked to a halt and I could hear the music again. My gurney rumbled off the elevator and was wheeled over to the nearby Nurse's station.

The capturing Nurse gave my medical chart to the Nurse standing behind the station's high counter. They chatted for a moment then the Nurse came back over and said goodbye to my parents and wished me a speedy recovery. She took the next elevator down and I never saw her again.

My parents and I waited in silence for the Station Nurse to finish reading my chart. A hidden transistor radio was softly playing The Beatles newest hit 'All you need is Love'. The Station Nurse finally put down my chart "You're in luck, a bed's available, we'll have it ready soon."

She stepped out from behind the counter. Boy was she short. I noticed she was dressed in a white shirt and skirt, a white belt, white shoes with a starched white cap on the crown of her head.

She wheeled me down the hall past dark rooms with ½ open doors. A painful, sorrowful moan escaped from one room as we passed. It heightened my anxiety. Half way down the hall the Station Nurse pushed my gurney against the wall across from my room.

The whole time, my parents never left my side. My Mom kept holding my hand and telling me everything was going to be okay, that I'd feel better after a good night's sleep.

A few quiet moments later two Nurses came down the hall. They wheeled my gurney through the enormous door into my new room and lifted me onto the bed.

It was excruciatingly uncomfortable, more torture device than bed. The mattress was thin, lumpy and plastic coated, as were the pillows. The starched arctic white sheets were stiff and ill fitting. The bed's metal frame and springs creaked and moaned whenever I moved. However the bed was electric. With the press of a button I could raise my head, or feet, or both. Maybe I could find a more comfortable position if I played with it a little.

Playing with the bed would have to wait as the two Nurses tucked me in. Then they gave my parents a comforting nod and left. Moments later a Doctor and Nurse arrived wheeling a cart of supplies up to the side of my bed. The Nurse smiled at me, but they worked in silence.

Long thin needles were inserted into the backs of both my hands, just below the wrist. The Nurse guided these needles up into the veins of my forearms. The end of the needle sticking out of my hands had a blue plastic cap. This cap was designed so the intravenous tubes could be attached or detached without removing & reinserting the needle. The needles were taped in place. The rubber tops of glass bottles of antibiotics were pierced by needles and hung upside down from two stainless steel poles affixed to my bed frame. Clear rubber tubes connected the needles in the bottles to the needles in my hands. With the turn of its tiny wheel a small plastic device straddling each tube, controlled the rate the drops of antibiotic flowed down the tubes.

The Doctor set the antibiotic drip rate while the Nurse taped my hands & forearms to flat stiff boards. I could still move my arms, but couldn't grab anything. When I asked why, the Doctor told me it was to keep me from accidently tearing out the intravenous while I slept.

The Nurse reached under my gown and applied several sticky pads to my chest. Then she attached wires, which ran to a heart monitoring machine.

Finally, an oxygen tent was brought in and set up. It covered me from head to waist. Its clear plastic was supported by a thin metal framework which allowed the Nurses to reach in, but didn't let the oxygen out. The crinkled clear plastic distorted sight and sound.

Before she left, the Nurse raised the metal side rails of the bed, locking them in place heightening my feelings of imprisonment.

"Why do you have to raise the rails?" I asked. "So you won't fall out of bed while you're sleeping," she whispered reassuringly. It did not have the desired effect.

The Doctor talked to my parents quietly then turned to me and said "I'll check in on you tomorrow, get some sleep," and left.

The Nurse stayed behind and tucked in my bed sheets while telling my parents visiting hours were over and please not to stay too long. Then she said good night and turned off the room's overhead lights as she left.

My parents came over to my bedside and promised to visit as often as possible. My Dad lifted the plastic tent and they both kissed me, bid a teary goodnight and left. My Dad with his arm around my mother's shoulder.

I was alone.

I tried to sleep in the strange bed, but couldn't roll over or get comfortable with all the tubes and wires connected to me. I was afraid of pulling something loose if I moved, even to scratch my nose.

Sleeping solely on my back was an unnatural position for me. Plus the plastic mattress & pillow heated up if I lay in one position too long.

I slept badly, waking every so often to have a coughing fit, or when the flashlight wielding Guard Nurse made her hourly rounds. I was regularly startled awake wondering "Where am I? Who's there? What do they want?"

The distortion caused by the thick plastic of the oxygen tent confused my tired mind for a second until my memory woke up. Then I'd ask the annoying Nurse what time it was and try to go back to sleep. That proved difficult with the unnerving sounds of the other patient's moans, groans & coughs filling the night.

Then, near morning, a Nurse I'd never seen before tiptoed quietly into my room. She wheeled an almost silent cart full of test tubes, needles, etc. in front of her. She skillfully maneuvered it around my bed in the dim light of my room.

"I'm so sorry. I have to wake you…" she looked at a list on the top of the cart,"…David." She went on to explain that she was from the Lab downstairs, here to draw blood. This was going to become part of my daily routine while in Hospital.

Still half asleep when she swabbed my inner elbow with alcohol, I came full awake when she stuck a big needle in my left arm and drew three vials of blood.

It hurt a little, but I was used to needles, having taken one a day for the past four years. The Vampire Nurse as I called her, told me I was a brave boy and to go back to sleep. My blood was sent to the Lab in the Hospital basement for analysis and to check my blood sugars.

The glucometers Diabetics use today to get their blood sugar readings in five seconds wouldn't be invented for another twenty years. My blood, drawn at dawn, took a couple of hours to test, and another hour for the results to be delivered to my floor. My sugars were high to begin with due to the infection and lack of exercise.

I was fed intravenously for a couple of days. My appetite finally came back one morning. I asked a Nurse for something to eat while she was giving me my morning injection. "Well, you must be feeling better if you got your appetite back," she beamed, adding "If the Doctor says it's Okay you'll probably get lunch." That sounded promising to me.

The Doctor made his rounds every day about the same time, between 9 and 11 am. I was starving by the time he got there. After tapping my chest and back, listening to my breathing through his stethoscope, peering down my throat, checking my chart and asking me how I felt, he pronounced me fit to eat and left. The attending Nurse smiled and went off to order me a lunch.

I sat in anxious anticipation of the meal trolley for over an hour. An eternity for a starving 9 year old boy. I listened intently for the sound of the trolley as it was pushed over the gap between elevator and our floor. A loud distinct clattering as dozens of trays, cutlery, and food laden plates were bounced around inside. That sound was like ringing the dinner bell for us patients.

After what seemed like hours I heard the elevator's Bing and the trolley's clattering. I followed its sounds as it slowly made its way down the hall, finally stopping outside my room. I heard a tray being slid out. "Is that one mine, did I get one?" I fretted.

A second later a silent, nameless, faceless, hair capped, member of the kitchen staff entered carrying my lunch on a plastic tray. I adjusted the bed and slid down into a sitting position. My lunch tray was placed on my bedside table which was then cranked up & moved into place so I could eat lunch in bed.

The cutlery was stainless steel, the white dishes, ceramic. The main course was hidden under a stainless steel cover. I was drooling by this point.

I lifted the lid…2 pieces of bread, a pad of butter on a tiny, thin square of wax cardboard with a wax paper cover. 2 packaged sticks of cheddar cheese. A covered bowl of what turned out to be chicken broth with a package of saltines on the side.

For dessert there was ice cream in a Styrofoam cup with a pull off cardboard lid. The lid was blue for vanilla. Pulling off the lid I noticed the ice cream in the middle was still frozen but the edge had melted into cream.

I devoured the entire meal in seconds, then had to stare at the bare tray until the kitchen staff came and silently removed it exactly half an hour later.

A few days on the strict hospital diet and my blood sugars levelled out, but it felt like I was eating half what I needed. Didn't they realize I was a growing boy?

After lunch, there was nothing much to do, so I played with the bed's remote control settings raising my head and back into a sitting position. As my head rose, my bum slid down the bed until my feet hit the footboard & stopped me. From this uncomfortable sitting position I passed the time listening and taking in my surroundings.

My room had crème colored walls with one big window to my right. The ceiling was flat white with a fluorescent tube light over my bed and the empty bed beside mine. The floors were tile, a speckled black, gray and white pattern. They were one meter by one meter, separated by a thin strip of stainless steel. A curb, two inches high and six inches wide, ran along the bottom of the room's walls. There was a bathroom in the room, but it may as well have been on Mars for all the good it was to me those first few days. The nurses brought me a cold silver bedpan whenever I needed to do my business.

I watched the heart monitor, wondering if I could affect the readings by slowing my breathing and relaxing. Like the Yogi I'd recently seen on a documentary about bio feedback. I concentrated and sure enough my heart rate slowed. Cool! I slowed it so much in fact that it set off the alarm. A Nurse promptly came to reset the machine. I could also raise my heart rate by breathing faster and concentrating on an angry memory. It passed some of the vast span of time between tests, meals and visits from the outside world.

My parents took turns visiting me daily for the first week. My brother and sister weren't allowed to visit me in the Hospital. They were too young. I remember my parents gave me reports of their successes, hijinks and crayoned pictures of the whole family together and happy, with "Get Well" and "Come Home Soon" scrawled across them. I missed them terribly.

A couple of days after being admitted the oxygen tent was removed. My parents began to visit a little less frequently once I was out of the tent. By the end of the first week one of my arms was released from the board and intravenous. The wires connected to the sticky pads on my chest and under my arm were disconnected. Now I could get out of bed and with my bottle of antibiotics on a pole on wheels, move around the room, go to the bathroom in something other than a cold bed pan.

After ten days I was freed of the intravenous completely and allowed to leave my room. I was playing in front of the Nurse's station when an elevator went Bing and the meal trolley came clattering off. I hadn't actually seen the trolley until then.

It looked like a tall shiny silver box on wheels. Made of stainless steel it stood 5' high x 4' long x 2' wide. I dared to touch the side of it once, it was very warm, almost hot. The doors at its narrow ends were open so the trays could be quickly & easily removed.

I peeked inside and counted 40 meal trays. I saw bowls of Jello squares and was tempted to steal one, but there were too many people around and I knew it was wrong.

After waiting hungrily for each meal to arrive, day after day, week after week, I became conditioned. Whenever I heard the meal trolley's clattering sound I'd start salivating like Pavlov's dog.

Fresca and TAB were introduced to me one day when I asked a Nurse for something to drink. These were the first carbonated soft drinks for Diabetics. They tasted horrible. Fresca was a cloudy light green drink that had a metallic citrus aftertaste.

TAB was the sugar free equivalent of Coke. It was brown, carbonated, and tasted a little like Coke, but with that metallic aftertaste.

I got used to their aftertaste over time, drinking them happily as a change from water, juice, or milk. In 1967, there were very few sugar free candies, gum, pop, cookies etc. and they all tasted like cheap copies of the original treat.

To prevent me from getting bored or homesick, my Dad brought me books and Plasticine. He also picked up the coolest plastic Dinosaurs in the Hospital lobby gift shop, whenever he came to visit. He knew some of their names and encouraged me to discover the names of the others by borrowing dinosaur books from the book cart which was wheeled into my room once a day.

My parents started visiting every other day, and only one of them came. It was getting too expensive for a baby sitter for my brother and sister. My parents drove an hour each way to visit me for an hour, sometimes less, but they knew those visits meant everything to me. Without them, I was cut off from the rest of the world.

Dad started giving me a couple of dollars whenever he visited. He talked to the Nurses and arranged it so I'd be allowed to go down to the Hospital Gift Shop to buy a toy or comic, as long as a Nurse escorted me.

I went to the store a couple of times. The Nurses seemed to love taking me there, and I loved the change of scenery. I was young, inquisitive and full of energy once I started to really feel better.

I was in grade four at the time, but hadn't thought about school since being admitted. There was plenty of stuff for me to learn in the Hospital. Everyone there knew about Diabetes. Back home, I was the only Diabetic attending my public school. Although I kept it well hidden, every once in awhile I'd have a reaction in class. It drew everyone's attention all the sweating and confusion. I'd be taken to the Nurses office where she'd give me a Styrofoam cup of Orange juice and several sugar cubes. I'd sit there crunching sugar and drinking juice until I felt better, then back to class I went.

Most of the students of Clifton Public School lived within walking distance and went home for lunch.

While I was in the Hospital, a cute classmate named Lindsey Stone did my homework for me during her lunches. Not only was she nice enough to volunteer to help me, but she was smart enough to get me great marks.

In the Hospital I had 24 hour a day attention. I was fed, bathed & clothed. Surrounded by intelligent, caring Hospital staff and visited regularly by loved ones.

Yet a gilded cage is still a cage and I longed for freedom. I started asking my parents when I could go home. They said, "When the Doctors says you can." I heard that line so often I began to think they didn't want me to come home. Maybe I'd done something wrong.

Staying in the Hospital became like staying in prison. The Nurses were the Guards, my Doctor the Warden. I tried sweet talking him, promising him I'd be good at home. I told him I got more exercise at home so my sugars would be better there etc., anything to get him to release me. But every time I asked when I was going home he just said "A couple more days."

My Dad pointed out all these great things to make my stay more bearable. But kids never react the way you think they will once you leave the room.

I took my Dad's words to heart and tried to look at my stay as a spa vacation. I read books and magazine articles on the subjects I wanted to know about: Dinosaurs, the human body, geography, Comic heroes, etc.

The hospital had a pool and Arts and Crafts classes. I made a stuffed squirrel, cut from felt using a pattern and stitched together by yours truly. I wove a basket one day, but once I found out about paint by numbers and doodle art that was how I spent a lot of my time.

It really wasn't too bad. By the end of the second week I felt much better and honestly believed I was ready to go home.

Then one eventful day, I was taken to the Lab in the Hospital basement for blood work. During the elevator ride back up to my floor, we stopped on the second floor. I'd never been to the second floor before.

When the elevator doors opened, the chaotic sounds and tantalizing smells of the Hospital's Cafeteria flooded in. Clattering dishes and cutlery, the cash register ringing, the background buzz of dozens of staff conversations all taking place at once.

The smell of baked goods, fruit juices and main course meals made my mouth water. By leaning forward I could see the register from the elevator, and noticed chocolate bars and other forbidden sweet treats there. Then some people got on and pressed the buttons to their floors. I decided to come explore this floor a bit more.

To be painfully honest, I probably would have been released in a couple days tops, if I hadn't succumbed to temptation.

I was allowed to play in the main hall outside my room as long as I didn't get in the way. I learned to stay on the raised curb that ran down both sides of the hall. The curbs made an excellent out of the way place for me to play with my plastic dinosaurs and still watch the goings on of the hospital.

As the days passed the chaotic hustle and bustle of Nurses, Janitors, Visitors, Doctors, patient admissions & discharges, meals & meds, staff breaks & shift changes, night wakings and dawn blood drawings, all became part of my floor's daily routine.

I figured out when I could play quietly outside my room and when I could take off unobserved and explore other parts of the Hospital. Once or twice I even peaked into other patient's rooms on other floors. I was caught wandering other floors several times. I explained that I was bored and they'd tell me to go back to my floor before the Nurses got worried.

Once while I was wandering, a Nurse introduced me to a boy in a wheelchair. He could put both his feet behind his head without using his hands. He was also the first person I ever saw balance his wheelchair on two wheels, spin it in place , then take off down the hall, stopping just before hitting the door at the end.

I was a stranger in a strange land, but no longer bored. After a few minutes of wandering a Nurse would always come along, check my wristband, and ask me to return to my own floor.

I can recall only one cellmate, a pleasant teenage boy with Haemophilia. We shared the room for about a week. He had a big stack of Marvel Super Hero comics. He shared his comics with me. I was introduced to the Fantastic 4, the Hulk, the Green Lantern and many more. Whenever those heroes were imprisoned like me, they'd figure a clever way of using their super abilities and will power to escape their captors. It passed the time and gave me inspiration.

My cellmate was no problem, I'd duck out when his parents came to visit. I'd return before they left so they didn't miss me.

The Nurses kept a casual eye on me while I played in the hall. I'd become such a regular sight, I was practically invisible. I discovered that if I only vanished for a few minutes at a time nobody missed me. I could leave my floor and go where I pleased.

The next day I played down the hall, closer and closer to the door leading to the stairs, timing my escape. At the door I did a quick check to make sure nobody was watching.

I pushed the thumb latch down silently & opened the door just enough to squeeze through. Then I grabbed the handle so the self-closing door wouldn't make the tell-tale click clack sound alerting any curious Nurses within earshot.

I put the toys I'd been playing with behind the door, planning to pick them up when I came back. I ran down seven flights of stairs, past doors with their floor's number stenciled on the back.

I wasn't used to so much exercise, arriving at the second floor rather breathless, but excited. In the Cafeteria, I picked a ½ Moon and an Oh Henry bar, paid for them and headed for the stairs. So far so good. Halfway back up to my floor, I stopped and sat on a step to sample these forbidden foods. After the first sweet, fluffy, bite, I devoured the entire ½ Moon. I'd never had anything like it before. It was decadently sweet.

I had no idea what was going to happen. Then, nothing happened, I didn't die, and nobody caught me. Only trouble was, I wanted more, but if I didn't get back upstairs soon I'd be missed.

I almost risked it, but when I heard a stairway door open on the floor below me I took off like a scared rabbit. I leapt up the stairs two at a time enjoying the stimulating sugar rush. Reaching my floor, I scooped up my toys and opened the door a crack, just enough to see if anyone was looking my way. It looked clear enough, so I innocently meandered and played my way back to my room.

I got away with this crime for a couple of weeks and was so proud of myself. I was getting away with murder. I just didn't realize at the time that it was my own murder I was getting away with.

The extra butter tarts, chocolate bars & candies on top of my diet raised my sugars. The Doctors tried to increase my insulin thinking it was still the pneumonia affecting my sugars. Maybe I'd have to take a bit more insulin from now on.

They also increased my activity level. I went for walks and swims, took activity classes like basket weaving, clay sculpting and stuffed animal making. Although all this extra attention and activity cramped my style a bit I still found time to hit the cafeteria once a day.

With my sugars rising daily, my personality slowly changed. I became much more melancholy. I was waiting impatiently for the meal trolley hours before it came. I drank pitchers of water. When my parents visited, all I wanted to talk about was getting out & going home. They tried to explain to me that my sugars were still too high, that the Doctors had to get them under control before they could let me go home safely. My parents obviously didn't love me.

The next day, as usual, my Doctor, with several Interns in tow, entered my room. He introduced me to the group as usual, asked me how I felt, as usual, checked my chart inside the metal clipboard at the foot of my bed, as usual. This was part of the daily routine. So much so that after a week I thought about asking the Doctor how he was.

One morning when he asked if I had any questions, instead of my usual "No," I surprised him by asking how he was, and of course when I could go home? The interns chuckled at my questions. My Doctor said, "As soon as your sugars come down, we'll see, maybe in a couple of days." Translation to an nine year old cheating Diabetic: "Never."

I grew bolder as the days passed. Idle hands are the tools of the devil, as the saying goes. I kept hitting the caf and the Doctors kept increasing my insulin dosage, playing catch up with my unexplainable rising sugars. This went on for a week.

I was becoming a bothersome problem for my Doctors. They couldn't figure out why my sugars weren't coming down, in fact they were heading in the opposite direction. It defied all logic.

They increased my blood sugar testing, trying to identify when my sugars spiked. One day the Lab Nurse came and took blood from my arm a total of thirteen times. I looked like a junkie with needle tracks up both arms and felt like a human pin cushion by the end of the day.

They seemed to be making a big deal about my blood sugar test results, so I started asking them what they were. The Nurses saw no harm so they told me. Day after day the numbers climbed.

Every day I asked my Doctor, "Can I go home today?" He kept giving evasive answers like, "When your sugars are under control, maybe tomorrow." With my habitual cheating, I knew that wasn't going to happen anytime soon.

I kept begging my parents to get me out of there. Every time they visited, I pleaded, cried and wailed for them to take me with them when they left. I cried rivers, cursed them, swore I'd never love them again and threw childish tantrums when they went to leave, unable to take any more. I'd even hang onto one of their legs so they'd have to drag me along at least to the elevators, wailing all the way "Don't leave me, I'll be good!" They went home in tears more than once.

I couldn't help myself. My prolonged high sugars were messing with my emotions and personality. Well, that and the tediousness of Hospital life were making me crazy. A Dr. Jekyll and Mr. Hyde transformation occurred to an otherwise rational, happy child.

That's when I discovered that emotions can affect blood sugars the way blood sugars affect emotions. Negative emotions like hate, anger, frustration, sadness, etc., raise sugars. Positive emotions like love, serenity, satisfaction, happiness, etc., lower sugars. In the case of Diabetes, laughter really is the best medicine.

Well some genius must have figured out my secret cafeteria visits. In the fourth week of my stay a rogue Nurse from another floor caught me on the stairs.

I was sitting there eating a Vachon pastry when the door to the floor above where I was sitting opened. Footsteps started coming down the stairs. They were too close for me to escape, so I decided to bluff it through. I sat there with the smoking gun in my hand hoping beyond reason that the person about to discover me wasn't a Nurse or Doctor. That they'd just casually walk on by, ignoring me and my sinful crime.

Unfortunately it was a Nurse, who not only didn't walk on by she stopped beside me. I remember thinking "I am in so much trouble." Fear froze my brain. She innocently asked me what I was doing down here. I hadn't expected to be caught, so I had no answer. Instead, I blushed with guilty embarrassment and hung my head in shame. She took my hand and examined my hospital wrist band. It clearly stated I was a Diabetic. Busted! She looked at the pastry crusted around my mouth and her whole personality changed.

Deep down I knew such a good thing couldn't last, but I wasn't prepared for it to end so badly. The arresting Nurse hauled my sorry ass up to the Nurse's station on my floor. She didn't even let me stop to grab my dinosaurs from behind the stairwell door on the way.

We stood at the Nurse's station while she asked who was supposed to be watching me. There was quite a stink about how I'd been able to get by the entire Nursing staff , go downstairs and buy a Vachon from the caf.

There was an even bigger stink when I somewhat boastfully told them how long I'd been doing it. So with egg all over their faces, a Nurse went to call my parents. I pleaded with the remaining Nurse not to call my parents, but she just kept saying they had to.

I lived in fear of my parent's next visit. As the appointed hour approached I tried to think of something to say, something to justify my actions. I was clutching at straws, deluding myself. After all I had spent my allowance on food instead of toys, maybe they'd praise me for being so practical, but no such luck.

When my parents arrived, they didn't come over and give me a kiss like they always did. This was going to be bad. Instead, they took off their coats, hung them up and sat down beside my bed.

My father scolded me for lying. My mother expressed her disappointment in me for cheating on my diet. My father scolded me for fooling the Nurses and getting them in trouble. My mother asked, "Why?" It was like tag team scolding. By the end of their visit I felt like my parents would never trust me again. I'd sinned a great sin, committed an ignoble act. I was disgraced.

As punishment, I was sentenced to room arrest. No allowance. No playing in the halls. No leaving the floor without a Nurse. I was in solitary confinement. I couldn't even wait in the hall outside my room for the meal trolley.

Every time I stepped out of my room, at least one of the Nurses gave me the evil eye. I swear, if they'd been armed there'd have been many a warning shot whizzing by my head. Can you blame them? It was a harsh lesson but I learned how important staying on my diet was. My will power, patience and discipline were put to the test.

I spent the rest of my stay reading. Once a day the book cart was brought around by a volunteer. I read the Hardy Boys, National Geographic, anything to do with dinosaurs, or history. I was soaking up knowledge like a sponge.

Now when my parents visited we'd talk about what I'd read, not when I was leaving. My Dad always embellished what I'd read with something he'd read on that subject, didn't matter what subject. My father was a brilliant man.

After a week in solitary, adhering to my diet, and tinkering with my insulin dosages, my sugars did finally level out. After six exciting weeks, I'd earned my walking papers and was discharged with a stern warning not to cheat or I'd end up right back in the Hospital.

I don't think the Nurses were sad to see me go, the naughty Diabetic kid that caused so much trouble. Although they did all stop in to say goodbye and remind me to behave myself from now on.

Walking out of the Hospital, hand in hand with my parents, was like being released from prison. I was so proud and happy, I almost cried. I was just a little older, but a lot wiser. Now all I had to do was stick to my diet for the rest of my life and I'd be fine.

Piece of cake.

Ummmmm, cake.

Chapter 4
The Silent Treatment

With the back of his surgically gloved hand, Dr. Luke Cameron brushed aside the annoying shock of dark auburn hair that kept falling across his forehead. He held a cotton ball doused with alcohol in that hand. In his other gloved hand he held a ¾ full old fashioned glass syringe with a long needle. He was sitting in an uncomfortable wooden chair, keen to finish the treatment and get away from this annoying patient, Mr. Rob Burnett.

The two men sat silently in the kitchen of Mr. Burnett's rustic log cabin. He'd built it himself because he didn't trust anyone else to do it right. His cabin sat right smack dab in the middle of a hundred acres of sugar maple forest, deep in the heart of Muskoka.

Mr. Burnett sat with an elbow on the table, the other arm held out for an injection, shirt sleeve rolled up past his elbow. Without a word Dr. Cameron gave his patient's exposed inner elbow a single swipe with the cotton ball. Then painlessly slipped the long needle under the man's skin and into the vein, like he'd done it a thousand times before.

"A thousand!? Could this skeptical young man truly be the one thousandth Diabetic I've cured? Where does the time go?" Luke reflected as he finished the injection. Then deftly withdrew the needle, applied a dry cotton ball and bent Mr. Burnett's arm up in one fluid motion.

"There Mr. Burnett, now you just hold it like that for a few seconds while I get some tape from my bag," advised Dr. Cameron casually. He turned away and capped the needle of the glass syringe.

Then he reached over and opened his authentic nineteenth century black leather Dr. bag sitting on the table.

His bag was the kind Doctors had carried when they still made house calls. His wife Chloe had purchased it at an estate auction, several years back. From the moment he'd laid eyes on it he'd loved it, and had been travelling with it ever since. Luke thought it looked cool.

"That's it?" asked Rob Burnett dubiously. "One shot, Bam! I'm cured?"

"No, no, as I explained after last night's seminar, it'll take about twelve hours for the cure to take full effect. Then you'll be free to live your life without needles, pills or blood sugar tests. All you'll have to do to remain Diabetes free is eat a balanced diet, exercise daily, and get enough sleep."

As he spoke Dr. Cameron reached into his black bag and pulled out what looked to be a metal cigar tube. His long fingers nimbly removed its rubber cap, slipped the used needle into it and resealed it before replacing it gently into his bag.

This time when he withdrew his hand he was holding a roll of medical tape, scissors & a worn, leather bound journal. He laid it all out on the kitchen table as though he were preparing for surgery.

He straightened out Mr. Burnett's arm and taped the cotton ball in place. "You can take this off in a couple of hours, but I wouldn't lift anything heavy for the rest of the day if I were you. That could cause the injection site to bruise or bleed."

Then he put the tape & scissors back into his bag, removed his gloves and tossed them in too. Rob watched him tidy up. When he was finished there was no evidence he'd ever visited.

"How much did you say I owe ya for this Doc?" questioned Mr. Burnett.

"Well, if you want to give me something, give me your word you won't tell a soul about being cured. Just keep on with your regular life like you said you would at the seminar last night. Confidentially, that *is* why you were chosen to be cured in the first place."

"If this cure of yours really works, I won't breathe a word. Ain't nobody's business but mine. But if anything goes wrong, say this here cure of yours don't work like you say it will, I'll come looking for you and I won't be quiet about it. I'll bring the Police."

Luke Cameron's calm iridescent blue eyes stared back at Mr. Burnett. They didn't show his anger at being threatened, or the disdain he felt for anyone who'd take his cure then thank him with insults and threats. In Luke's ledger, Mr. Burnett now had two strikes against him.

Unfortunately this wasn't the first rude skeptic he'd run across, probably wouldn't be the last. Luke knew from experience that even the most jaded skeptics had changed their tune after experiencing the freedom of being cured, of being normal again. So he'd tolerate this ingrate's remarks in silence for now and just stared calmly at Mr. Burnett.

Rob Burnett found those eyes unsettling. He couldn't gauge the Doc's reaction to his warning in those two cold blue diamonds. They looked unnatural, which troubled Rob.

"You sure mine are gonna change too?" he asked, gesturing rapidly between his eyes and the Doc's with his index finger.

"Pretty sure, it's happened to everybody I've cured so far" replied Dr. Cameron.

"Hmm, guess it's better than taking needles every day, but it'll take some getting used to." Rob gave a half-hearted grin to mask the depth of his disappointment. All the girls in town liked his dark brown eyes, finding them mysterious and sexy.

"I'll have to think of something to tell the boys at work when they notice I got shiny blue eyes like you" worried Rob aloud. He didn't want to start lying to his friends. He wasn't very good at it.

Dr. Cameron had helped other patients hide or come up with an explanation for their blue eyes in the past, so he offered a solution. "Tell them it's a side effect to laser eye surgery, or new eye drops you're using. Just don't mention the cure."

"I won't," said Rob testily, "but I gotta give ya something for curin me Doc. Even if it ain't as much as you think it should be."

"Fine, if you feel that strongly about it, give me something before I leave next week."

"Like what?" asked Rob not wanting to insult the Doc with too cheap a gift.

"Whatever, me and the family are travelling, so just don't make it anything too big. How about I stop by next Wednesday and do a follow up. You can pay me then, Okay?"

"Fine, fine Doc" Rob reluctantly agreed, still not convinced this cure wasn't some sort of scam.

Luke had discovered early in his crusade that when he left payment for his treatment up to his patients, they tended to pay more than he would have charged. He'd already received so much from past patients that there was no reason to charge Mr. Burnett. Except to make him pay for his rudeness, and that was a good enough reason for Luke.

He adjusted his round wire framed glasses and opened his journal to the bookmarked page. Across the top of the page was Mr. Burnett's name and file #, beautifully written in Sanskrit. Sure enough Mr. Burnett was the 1000th Diabetic he'd treated. Dr. Cameron added the injection date and time beneath.

By his calculations, he'd cured one Diabetic for every day he and his family had been on the run. Not bad for a family guy hiding from the world's largest pharmaceutical company. Luke patted himself on the back with deep satisfaction. He closed his journal, reflexively patting it twice, then stretched an elastic band around it and gently placed it in his bag.

Then having neither need nor desire to remain in Mr. Burnett's company another minute, Dr. Cameron closed his bag, grabbed it by its comfortable handle and rose to leave. "Well Mr. Burnett, I really must be going now, several more house calls to make & Diabetics to cure today." He smiled and headed for the front door.

Rob Burnett nodded and followed Dr. Cameron to the door then curtly shook his hand, grudgingly saying "Thanks Doc. If this cure of yours really works, I'll keep your secret til the day I die."

Dr. Cameron tipped his head in gratitude, turned and walked over to his bicycle. It was leaning against the closest of the Maple trees lining Mr. Burnett's ½ km long driveway. He slipped his black bag into the carrying case on the back of his bicycle securing it with two bungee cords. He pushed off and peddled down the long gravel driveway without another thought of Mr. Burnett.

At the end of the winding driveway he stopped and rechecked the house calls route map his son Jim had made for him to follow. According to the map his next house call was to the right and about an hour's ride so he'd be getting there about lunch time, perfect.

He recalled as a Diabetic worrying about having a low blood sugar reaction due to all the riding he was doing, in the middle of nowhere and before a meal to boot. Now, as a normal person, he could enjoy the ride in the country, work up an appetite and if Mrs. Roberta Greene was true to her word, she'd have had a lunch prepared & waiting when he arrived.

As he rode along the lightly travelled gravel side road, he thought about the events that had led him here.

It all started while he was still attending Sir Craig Ventner's Institute of Advanced Genetics. He'd made several brilliant breakthroughs in his final year which had drawn the attention of the world's largest pharmaceutical companies.

Global Pharm was the most dominant, tendrils into every country on the planet, one point nine trillion dollars in annual revenue, centuries old and still growing. It was a monster.

One of their newest 'Reps', Jen Hanson, had been given Dr. Luke Cameron's recruitment as her first assignment. 'Rep' was the title given to drug company security agents. Reps protected the profitability, viability and necessity of the world's Pharmaceutical industry by any and all means necessary.

Jen was young, attractive & ambitious. Although she'd only been a Rep for a year she'd managed to be promoted several times. All the way up to recruitment level.

Recruitment bonuses and trailer fees added up to a small fortune at this level. This was her dream job and Luke Cameron was going to be her first recruit & first fortune. She had a good feeling about him when she examined his dossier.

Luke had two other lucrative job offers lined up, but Jen had seduced him before his meetings with her competitors. She'd gone so far as to spike his drink before she'd made him sign the contracts. Jen was attracted to Luke and decided to spend a wild night with him to celebrate her victory.

Early the next morning Luke had woken up to find his signature on every page of Global Pharm's iron clad contract. He couldn't remember signing them, and trying to remember just made his head hurt worse. So Luke had quietly got dressed, grabbed a copy of the contract and left without waking her. He felt used and unable to shake the feeling that he'd just sold his soul to the devil herself.

For the first few years at Global Pharm, he'd been satisfied, earning a fat salary with all the perks. His labs were state of the art, his team, enthusiastic and knowledgeable: Dr. Gustav Tavarich, Geneticist; Dr. Xiang Wa, Chemical Engineer; and Dr. Joanne Khan, Biologist. It was an esteemed group to be leading.

Even the projects they'd been assigned had been challenging and groundbreaking.

Jen had stayed in touch with him, even dropping by the lab periodically. She'd make small talk laced with suggestive comments and sexual innuendo. Luke had ignored her advances, once bitten, twice shy. Over time her uncomfortable visits became less frequent and finally stopped altogether to Luke's relief.

Then one day he and his team had been assigned a project that appeared to be half complete, which was odd. They'd always started from scratch before this. Luke figured out that it had been someone else's unfinished research notes and formulae to cure one of society's lesser-known fatal diseases.

His superior, Dr. Thadeus McKinnon, had ordered Luke's team to use the research to create a daily dose cure in pill or injection form for those with the disease. A sticky note had been attached to the instructions stating that a yearly vaccine would be acceptable, but a daily pill was preferred by the Board. Bonuses were promised, if they could accomplish their assignment by year's end.

His mind swam as he realized that he'd be allowed to continue doing research, but only to make sick people feel better for profit. Never to cure them.

Luke wasn't sure he could live with himself if he accepted this assignment. This was the first step on the slippery slope of moral compromise. He'd rushed out of the lab to clear his head and try to think this thing through.

After aimlessly wandering the streets for hours, he ended up at the coffee shop around the corner from his lab. That's where he ran into his high school sweetheart Chloe.

She was as beautiful & sweet as he remembered. Everything about her was generous and kind. They'd sat and talked as if the world around them had ceased to exist. Hours passed by unnoticed, until Chloe had glanced at her watch while reaching for her cup.

"Well would you look at the time. We've spent most of the day here. Won't they be upset with you at work?" she asked, genuinely concerned for his wellbeing.

"Yeah, I guess so. I don't really want to go back, but I am under contract and maybe I can still find a way to do some good."

They walked hand in hand to the coffee shop doors, natural as can be. Before parting, they excitedly made a date for dinner that night. Six months later they were married. Nine months after that they'd become parents of twins, Mark and Jade.

As Luke peddled along a particularly rough patch of road he had to dodge several rain filled potholes. The rough road reminded him of the first few years with Chloe. Not only had his conscience eaten away at him every day at the lab, but Chloe, Mark & Jade had developed Type 1 Diabetes. They'd learned to cope, but Luke felt useless.

He knew he had to find a way to work on a cure at Global Pharm's Labs, despite the strict rules and severe penalties against personal research projects. Luke had been forced to make the choice between his family and his career. That night at dinner he'd sworn to his family that he'd use all the Global Pharm resources at his command to find the cure for Diabetes.

The next day he'd asked Dr. McKinnon for extra lab time. Luke claimed he wasn't being stimulated enough by the assignments as of late. He wanted to conduct a few small experiments of his own.

Dr. McKinnon had looked him up and down. "Okay, Lab 327 just opened up, but for God's sake don't blow anything up. Keep me abreast of any discovery, and remember whatever you do discover, Global Pharm owns it. That's in your contract."

For the next couple of years Luke and his team worked evenings and Saturdays on his private project. They'd made several startling discoveries, keeping McKinnon apprised of most of them. A few they didn't. Those were the ones that crossed Global Pharm's 'do not pursue' research parameters.

Not completely satisfied with the number of discoveries he'd been made privy to, McKinnon spied on Luke and his team via surveillance cameras placed throughout the lab complex.

The Board of Directors at Global Pharm was made aware of Luke's cure research. Searching their historic data base for similar formulas, they discovered that Luke & his team were on the verge of recreating Dr. Fredrick Banting's cure for Diabetes.

Global Pharm was already an old company when Dr. Banting discovered the cure in 1918 during the first World War. His discovery had been purchased by Global Pharm before the public could be made aware of it. It was purchased for a mere ten million dollars, Banting's sworn silence and the promise of a Nobel Prize in exchange for developing his cure into something less permanent and more profitable. Something Diabetics would need to take once a day, a pill or injection.

After three more years of experimenting, Dr. Banting and his Global Pharm team developed Insulin. They conducted the first successful human trials in January 1922. Insulin met all of Global Pharm's requirements and in 1923 the Nobel Prize for Medicine was awarded to Dr. Banting.

Unfortunately, years later Dr. Banting had a change of heart after seeing the horrific complications brought on by long term use of Insulin. His guilt ate him up, ruined his marriage, ended his research and finally drove him to seek absolution by revealing to the world that a cure for Diabetes did exist. On his way to England to tell his story to a reporter named Franks, his plane mysteriously crashed over the Atlantic. His body was never found.

The Global Pharm Board of Directors had voted to assign Luke's team multiple projects aimed to bog them down and interfere with their cure research. If that didn't work then more drastic measures would have to be employed.

As he peddled along a stretch of sun dappled road he smiled, marvelling at how during all that, he and Chloe managed to find the time and energy to have two more children, Fran & Jim. Those had been fast, hard and rewarding years.

One day in June he'd complained to Chloe of constantly being tired & thirsty, so she'd tested his blood sugars. They'd been 13.4, confirming he had Diabetes too. He'd had a bit of trouble adjusting to the whole regimented lifestyle associated with good Diabetes care. Not to mention the challenges involved in hiding the symptoms of his high & low blood sugar reactions at work.

He couldn't inform his employers of his condition, that would mean immediate dismissal. It was common knowledge throughout the drug industry that a disease was as good as a pink slip. Luke needed to stay in that industry, at least until he'd cured his family. So he kept his illness a secret, even from his team and redoubled his efforts in the Lab.

Luke knew he realistically had eleven months to find the cure. That's when his next mandatory annual physical exam would be given by Global Pharm Doctors. Unless they were complete morons, he'd be discovered and dismissed.

As the months ticked by, Luke focused his team on their cure project, to the exclusion of many other assigned projects. It took them 10.5 months to finish it, but after almost a decade at Global Pharm, Dr. Cameron and his team formulated a potential cure.

With just 2 weeks before his physical, Luke conferred with his team about taking their formula straight to Phase II, animal trials, without their superior's approval or knowledge.

They all knew this was a grievous lapse in company law. But they were so close to proving their cure worked, that they threw caution to the wind and drove on.

Luke peddled a bit faster as he recalled the day they'd tried the first doses on a dozen white haired, pink eyed, lab rats. 12 hours after injection each rat's blood sugars were tested. They were all perfectly normal.

The team had all looked up from the results at the same time. For the briefest of seconds they'd stared at each other in silent shock. "Does this mean...?" asked Tavar in hushed disbelief? Then as one mighty chorus of almost hysterical voices they'd shouted, "We did it!"

Luke was the first to confirm aloud, their world altering discovery.

"We've cured Diabetes."

"Hallelujah," One of the team added happily.

"We're heroes!" another laughed.

"We're going to be famous!"

"And rich, don't forget the royalties alone are going to be astronomical."

"That's right, cause next year's Nobel Prize is in the bag, eh boys and girls?" added Dr. Tavarich, slapping Luke on the back.

"Three cheers for Dr. Cameron..." began Dr. Wa, but Dr. Khan interjected, "and his most excellent team."

Nodding a polite acknowledgement, Dr. Wa continued, "...discoverers of the Cure for Diabetes!" They'd shouted, "Hip Hip Hooray!" three times then exploded with elated laughter, hugging each other, slapping each other on the back and singing 'We are the Champions' by Queen.

Luke had wept with joy and relief. He'd picked up his latest favorite lab rat, looked it straight in its little pink eyes and said "Thank You Fred, thanks for saving my family."

Then it happened.

As Luke stared into Fred's beady little eyes, the rat's irises changed from pink to a startling iridescent blue. Fred's new eyes glittered back at Luke as he examined them from different angles. Luke had silenced his still celebrating team and held up Fred. "We have a problem." The team could see Fred's eyes glittering from across the room.

They'd run over to the cages and checked all the rats' eyes. One after another their eyes changed until every last one had glittering iridescent blue irises. Luke had the team retest every rat's blood sugars. The results were all 5.5. At least they'd remained normal, proving the cure did work, it just had a hell of a side effect.

Luke rode over a rough patch of gravel at the same time he recalled what happened next. Despite the obvious yet apparently harmless side effect, Luke had still been excited beyond reason. He'd immediately taken their amazing test results and the cured rat to his superior. McKinnon's written approval was necessary to take their cure to Phase III, Human trials. He'd been confident that McKinnon and the Board of Directors would quickly approve and produce an experimental batch of the cure. Luke's family were just months, perhaps weeks, away from being cured.

He'd barged past McKinnon's secretary and into his office, announcing proudly that he and his team had cured Diabetes! To his astonishment and dismay instead of praise and congratulations, McKinnon began ridiculing Luke. He was chastised for deviating from his assigned projects and not keeping him apprised of any progress, as they'd agreed.

"Global Pharm's labs are not for your personal experiments. Do you have any idea how many FDA, CDC, EPA, local and federal laws you've violated by taking this unsanctioned experiment this far!"

McKinnon had started banging his fist on his desktop as he spoke. Luke had never seen him act this way before. He didn't know what to say or do that wouldn't further enrage the man.

"I could lose my job over this too you know!" he interjected desperately, then continued berating Luke almost without a pause.

"You have willingly delayed the approved experiments you're being paid to turn into profitable medication for the world's sick and needy. You cannot spend this company's valuable resources on unprofitable experiments riddled with side effects. You're practically a traitor. At best you & your team are liabilities to this company and this industry," spat McKinnon.

It was at that very moment Luke had realized that his Cure may very well have killed his career.

Before Luke could say a word, the Chairman of the Board, Mr. D. C. Scollick, had entered McKinnon's office. He'd silently slipped through a side door that led directly to the Boardroom via a short hallway.

Mr. Scollick was a tall thin elderly man with brush cut steel grey hair, a clean shaven face and gold framed glasses. He wore an expensive looking dark blue tailored suit that made him appear to be all business. There was no trace of a smile upon his face, nor did it look like one had ever dared appear there. He told Luke, none too politely, to go wait outside until he was needed.

Sitting there under the secretary's evil glare, Luke tried to overhear what was being said, but had only heard muffled conversation until the Chairman's booming voice had rang out.

"Well, doesn't this genius of ours realize there's no profit in a cure...any cure."

McKinnon had said something, but Luke couldn't make it out.

"Well, we can't have him running around our labs doing whatever he wants, not on our time, with our money, no sir, we're running a business here," boomed Mr. Scollick.

Dr. McKinnon mumbled something again.

"No, no, Code Nine for Dr. Cameron immediately. That's the Board's final decision Thadeus," ordered Mr. Scollick. An ominous moment of silence had followed.

McKinnon's secretary's intercom buzzed loudly. She didn't answer it, she just stared at Luke dispassionately and pointed at the office doors.

Back in the office, Luke noticed the Chairman had left and McKinnon was hunched over his desk filling out forms. Without looking up from the papers McKinnon said, "Dr. Cameron your services will no longer be required." No sooner had the words left his lips than two big beefy security guards entered the office. "Escort Dr. Cameron from the building,"

McKinnon ordered, looking up just long enough to shoot an angry glance at the guards, but avoiding eye contact with Luke.

In the months that followed, Global Pharm. had Luke professionally discredited and black listed throughout the pharmaceutical industry. His research had been marked classified and archived according to company policy, never to see the light of day again. His team had been split up and reassigned to other more lucrative projects with tighter security.

Knowing he'd been so close to producing a cure for his family only to have it destroyed for lack of profitability, drove Luke to the verge of a nervous breakdown. For over a month he'd done nothing, except sleep and eat when he had to. He rarely spoke to his family. His shame at having failed them and utter hopelessness of ever curing them had stolen his voice.

Then one day while he was sitting & silently gazing out the kitchen window at nothing, he suddenly jumped up and shouted "I've got it!" I know what I have to do, what we need to do, Yahoo!! We're moving!"

Chloe had just stared at him praying he hadn't finally gone over the edge. The kids on the other hand couldn't have been happier. They'd come from all parts of the house when Luke had shouted. They jumped up and down full of questions, where? Why? When? How?

Two months later they'd sold their house. They moved out of the city and relocated to a small dairy farm, on the outskirts of a small town, half way across the country.

The town didn't have a doctor so Luke set up his medical practice specializing in Diabetes care. Soon he and his family had settled into their new community.

Yet Luke Cameron was a man with a plan. Relocation was just the first step towards his ultimate goal and he was dogged in his pursuit of it.

Over the last six months he'd spent every spare minute converting the milk analysis room of his barn into a laboratory for his experiments. Exactly one year after being fired from Global Pharm, Luke began to secretly continue his Cure research. He picked up where he and his team had left off, working well past midnight every night. Two years later, he had indeed rediscovered and perfected a simple, inexpensive cure for Diabetes.

This time when Fred Jr. was cured and his new blue irises started glittering, there was no hugging or back slapping, no talk of heroes, history or Nobel Prizes. No, this time there was just Luke and Fred Jr. who he returned to his cage. Luke had stood silently savoring the utter satisfaction of having finally attained his ultimate goal. He alone now wielded the power to save his beloved wife and children. Luke felt like a god.

By himself, Luke had created a universal cure for Diabetes, applicable to animal and human alike. So without delay he took his experiment to Phase III Human trial. He sat on the stool in front of his work bench, tested & recorded his blood sugars, then drew a syringe full of his Cure and injected himself. He'd used the glass syringe that had come with his medical bag. As he held the cotton ball over the injection site he realized that may have been the last needle he'd ever have to take. Luke sat back and smiled as a relaxing warmth spread throughout his body.

Twelve hours after the injection his blood sugars were 5.5, perfect. He'd done it! He'd cured Diabetes…again. Twenty minutes later he was washing up before announcing his discovery to his family when the side effect occurred.

He was looking at himself in the bathroom mirror when his irises changed from their natural hazel color to the glittering blue.

Luke gave an involuntary shudder as he recalled that moment. One minute he was looking at himself, the next a stranger was staring back curiously from the mirror.

The second he walked into the house, Chloe and family had immediately noticed his new eyes. Mark and Jade thought they looked cool and each wanted a pair. Fran and Jim on the other hand were scared at first, seeing their Daddy with a stranger's eyes. Only when they'd seen his familiar fatherly love for them in those glittering eyes had they run up and hugged him. Then the young ones had both taken a much closer look. Fran had even tried to poke one with her finger.

Suddenly everyone had started asking questions. Luke had told them of his discovery and the side effect, swearing them to secrecy. "If Global Pharm finds out you've cured Diabetes again they'll try to ruin you again, won't they?" asked Chloe. "Never mind Global Pharm, every drug company in the world will want our heads if news of this gets out" answered Luke.

Chloe was sweet, but a real fighter when it came to her family. She'd looked Luke straight in the eye and said "If that's what we're up against, then side effect or not, I think you'd better take this opportunity to cure us, now, don't you?" "I couldn't agree more" Luke had beamed and turning to the kids said, "Okay boys and girls, you heard your Mother, who wants to be cured first?" Luke had prepared just enough of the Cure to give everyone one injection.

They all tested their blood sugars before the injection that night. Chloe was within the normal range, but all the kids were a little on the high side. Mark was the highest at 14.2 ml/dl. Chloe had given him a disappointed glare. Little Fran pointed at him and gave him the *shame on you* sign with her index fingers.

"Don't worry son, somebody had to have the highest reading. Today it was you, tomorrow's going to be a whole new ballgame," reassured Luke, seeing the shame & disappointment in his son's eyes. Soon there'd be no testing at all and they'd have one less source of disappointment in all their lives.

The next morning they'd all woken up with iridescent blue irises. It caused some laughter around the breakfast table when Jade said they looked like a family of aliens, especially Jim, who had insisted on having his head shaved yesterday at the barber shop.

They'd all tested their blood sugars before breakfast. Their results were all 5.5 ml/dl, perfectly normal. Chloe took Luke's face in her hands and gently kissed him on the forehead. The kids all got up from the breakfast table crowding around their father for a group hug and a barrage of grateful kisses. Then Chloe had asked if they had to stay on their strict diet, or could she and Jade make a celebration breakfast.

"As long as everyone agrees to test their sugars as usual for the next few days, then I don't see any harm in having a breakfast worthy of being cured," responded Luke. He'd wanted to study as many aspects of the Cure as possible under controlled conditions. At the same time, he wanted his family to begin living normal lives.

Luke had insisted that for a couple of days they didn't leave the farm. He wanted everyone close in case of any unexpected side effects. He also didn't want the town's folk to notice their eyes and start asking questions. Not until he had more answers or found a way to hide their differences.

Jim was okay with that. After the alien comparison, he'd started wearing a baseball cap and sun glasses.

Jade on the other hand was desperate to go to town and show off her new eyes to her girlfriends.

Luke had kept them all busy with chores around the farm. That allowed him to examine how activity affected their blood sugars. He'd concluded that if they worked between meals they could eat pretty much what they wanted. Exercise was the key.

Every meal time was spent discussing what to do with the Cure.

Luke remembered how after only two days Mark had started acting like a typical teenager, eating what he wanted, when he wanted it and as much as he wanted. Six days after being cured his Diabetes had returned and he'd had to start taking Insulin injections again. Mark had been so ashamed at being Diabetic again that he tried to hide the fact. His irises had changed back to their normal color, but nobody noticed because they were all wearing sunglasses all the time except when they slept. It was only when he'd had a reaction before dinner one night that they all realized Mark had Diabetes again. The rest of the family members, who'd stayed active and ate regular meals, remained cured.

Luke was unsure what the result of a second dose of the Cure would do to his son but he had to try. Fortunately for Mark, the Cure worked on him a second time, but his irises developed thin dark blue outer rings. After that close call Mark stayed on his diet religiously.

Luke hadn't taken any chances and gave everyone another dose of the Cure. The results were unexpected. With a second dose they didn't even have to exercise and their blood sugars remained normal.

Still faced with the question of what to do with the cure, Luke asked for everyone's opinion. Little Fran spoke up first. "Hide it Daddy, don't tell anyone. Only use it for us if our Diabetes comes back." She had a sweet tooth and just knew her Diabetes would return like Mark's had. It was only a matter of time and temptation.

Jade piped in next. "I could make us an untraceable web page where we could sell the Cure. Once the news spreads, and trust me it will, we'll be rich." Jim jumped in to support the online idea. "Yeah Dad, let's go online. We'll tell the world & be famous."

Mark had a different plan. "Let's sell it to our Government's Ministry of Health. Then the drug companies won't be able to stop its distribution."

"The drug companies have their fingers in every government Mark," began Luke. "They have cyber divisions constantly monitoring the web for anything of interest to the drug industry, and this Cure will definitely be of immense interest to them. The moment we use the web, or any technology that can be traced, or tracked back to us, the cure is doomed.

Once we're discovered, the drug companies will discredit the Cure saying it's unapproved, unsafe, needs more study, has side effects, or whatever. If dissuading and misleading the public doesn't work, they'll tie up the Cure in the courts for decades, or until everyone forgets that there ever was a Cure," prophesized Luke.

"Yup, we're going to have to look at this problem in a whole new way if we want to cure people around the world," he concluded.

Chloe, who'd been silent up till this point, added her two cents. "Curing Diabetics around the world is a noble quest and I love you for your desires, so I suggest curing your own patients is as good a place to start as any. Who knows, maybe the ones you cure will help you find a way to cure the world safely one day."

Luke took Chloe's advice and after referencing his patient files compiled a list of twenty three Diabetics. From conversations with them, he knew there were others.

Those Diabetics went to Doctors in one of the nearby towns, or the big city nearly two hours away, but he couldn't access their e-health files, or so he thought.

Jade brought her impressive computer skills to bear by hacking the e-health data base for her father. She compiled a master list of all the town's Diabetics with their complete medical history. There were just fifty six names on that first list. The Cameron family knew most of them personally. It was a small town.

Luke's first instinct had been to cure everyone on the list, but as the family discussed the names on the list he realized it wouldn't be safe to cure everyone. He'd have to play God and choose which of his neighbours he'd cure and which ones he wouldn't.

As Luke skimmed over the list, some of the names jumped out at him. They were notorious gossips. Grabbing a pen he struck their names off the list as security risks.

So began the culling of his first list. If their medical records classified them as overweight or obese, he struck their names off. Anyone with a history of high blood sugars was off the list. If they suffered complications so severe they couldn't lead normal lives even if they were cured, with a heavy heart he struck them off the list as well. In the end just 12 names remained, most of which were unfamiliar to Luke and family.

They'd discussed how best to approach the people left on the list. Luke couldn't just walk up and say "Good morning Joe, I've discovered the Cure for Diabetes, want some?"

Chloe suggested that Dr. Cameron hold a private, Diabetics only, seminar about the latest in Diabetes research. "We'll invite the dozen Diabetics remaining on the list. At the seminar we'll have them fill out a screening questionnaire. Who you choose to cure can be based on their answers."

Luke thought it was a splendid idea and gave her a kiss of appreciation. What would he do without her? He couldn't bear to imagine. Then he gave each of his children a kiss and started working on a list of questions while Chloe got the children ready for bed.

That first seminar drew all twelve Diabetics, who'd completed the questionnaire. They'd listened to Luke speak and asked many questions afterwards. The next day Luke and family closely scrutinized the answers on their questionnaires. Two had been filled out as obvious attempts at humor, which the family enjoyed, but cost the comedians the Cure.

Most of the others had given answers that left the family or Luke with doubt. Fran came up with the rhyme "When in doubt cross them out," which sounded good to Luke and helped whittle down the list even further. In the end only three candidates met all Luke's criteria.

Udo Wadien: the town barber. His claim to fame was that he'd done hairstyling and special effects makeup for a B movie years back. He'd mention it to every customer as a conversation starter when he cut their hair. He'd also founded the local theatre group which put on two plays a year.

L.J. Savage: used car salesman, mechanic, avid camper and karaoke singer. At six feet nine inches, he had the distinction of being the tallest man in town. Second tallest in the county. He also owned one of the two used car lots in town, and worked as its head mechanic. He wasn't out to get rich he just liked working on motors.

Ms. Olga Kraft: famous around those parts as a great marathon cyclist. She'd won several trophies and awards in her last dozen races. She was sole owner of the 'Cycle of Life', the only bike shop in town. Her dream was to open a bike shop in every Province & Territory before she turned 30.

The next evening, *The Chosen*, as Mark liked to call them, were each paid a house call by Dr. Cameron. He told them he'd just been passing by and decided to drop by and discuss the answers they'd given on their questionnaire. Over the course of their conversation he'd asked each of them three simple questions.

"What would you give to be cured of Diabetes?" Each of the chosen had responded with, "Why, do you have a cure?" To which Luke just smiled and said "Yup."

Their shocked pause allowed Luke to ask the second question. "Once cured will you keep it secret?" Each one had asked him, "Why?" Luke had told them the whole truth, his past, the threat of the drug companies, the risk of redeveloping Diabetes, everything.

They had each swallowed hard as they grasped the fact that being cured had unimagined consequences and conditions. Luke had given them each a moment to absorb his story and agree or disagree to carry on. He still had one last secret to reveal and question to ask before he gave them their injections.

Udo, L.J. & Olga had each agreed to keep it secret and each asked if there were any more surprises. Luke had found that amusing. "Just one" he'd answered them "There's a side effect." As he spoke, he took off his dark glasses revealing his glittering blue eyes.

Then looking them straight in their amazed eyes he asked his final question. "Can you conceal the only known side effect to the cure?"

L.J. had exclaimed "Whoa, wait, that's it, sparkly blue eyes is the only side effect? Big deal. Cure me."

Olga had laughed and said "Cool," the way Jade and Mark had when they'd first seen them. "Do I *have* to hide them, they're so beautiful."

"I'm afraid so, right now it's too dangerous for any of us to be noticed." Luke had replied.

Olga had shrugged, smiled acceptingly and said "Oh well, it's a small price to pay. Cure me please."

Yet it was what Udo had said, upon seeing his startling eyes, that had really opened Luke's eyes. "What, gorgeous blue glittering eyes is the side effect? I love it! Doc, I have contact lenses in every color of the rainbow. My eyes are so dull, common really. So I started collecting colored lenses after I did that special effects driven Tex/Mex horror flic years back. Believe me when I tell you honestly, hiding these beauties will be no problemo. Hey, can I fix you up with a pair?"

"Got enough for me and my family, six pair in all?" asked Luke as an idea germinated in his mind. "Noah problemo Doc, I'll go get them, right after you cure me," Udo said smiling.

Luke had smiled back, injected, bandaged and advised him. Then he and Udo sat and had a long talk about hair and makeup.

After curing the first three of the Chosen, Luke discussed what to do next with his family.

After much heated debate, Mark suggested they take a long road trip, delivering the Cure cross-country by making house calls. "Like Doctors did in the old days of real medicine."

They all thought it was a great idea. Deciding to only make house calls in small towns and villages for security's sake. The big cities had too many cameras and tracking devices for them to remain off the drug company's grid for long. Staying unnoticed as long as possible would allow Luke time to cure whoever he chose.

Using Jade's access to e-health files, Luke had her compile lists of potential Diabetics in all the small towns and villages across the country. They'd visit the places with the most Diabetics first. That way he'd cure the most people in the shortest time.

As they began travelling and Luke had started curing people, Jade suggested changing their health records to show they never had Diabetes. For three years they'd been at it and they'd never looked back.

Luke looked back over his shoulder to see that there were no cars coming before crossing the road and coasting up to the wrought iron gates at the entrance to Ms. Roberta Green's estate. He hopped off his bike to admire the view through the gates. The mansion was at the end of a long winding driveway lined with tall majestic pines that filled the air with their scent.

Looking around Luke noticed that one of the enormous field stone pillars, to which the gates were hinged, had an intercom system. He walked his bike over and pressed the buzzer. Luke hoped the treatment went quickly, he was hungry and still had three more house calls to make that day. He had a schedule to keep, which included spending time with his family at the Busker Festival this town was famous for and be on the road by next Wednesday.

Four Days Later

Rob Burnett had only enjoyed his freedom from Diabetes for a couple of days before fate intervened. He was knocked unconscious at work and rushed to the nearby big city hospital that specialized in head injuries.

Dr. Weeber, the Emergency room Physician that day, pried open Rob's eyes to check pupil reaction. He actually gasped in surprise when he saw the iridescent blue pupils sparkling back at him. They were unnatural, but certainly not the result of a head injury. He examined the eyes closer, nope, not contact lenses. That narrows down the causes to an as yet unidentified chemical or drug reaction. Whatever it was, it most likely caused his patient's accident.

Dr. Weeber knew the drill regarding suspected drug reaction. First thing to do was notify the pharmaceutical company immediately. Maybe there was some new drug trial going on that he didn't know about. There seemed to be a lot of them lately and he didn't have time to read them all.

He grabbed one of the nurses and asked her to look for the drug company research & recall phone number. After a quick computer search the only number she could find was for Global Pharm's head office. She filled out their online drug trial information request form and sent it in under Dr. Weeber's name.

At Global Pharm, Dr. Weeber's request for information regarding drug trial side effects was quickly sent down to the Drug Testing & Recall department supervisor, Dr. Alex Price.

Not wanting to deal with it just before his holidays, he dumped the file on the desk of his newest lackey and pet Rep, Jen Hanson. She'd been demoted to the tedious job of intelligence gathering for Field Reps and Recruiting Reps. It was insulting, grunt work for a trained Rep like herself.

Her Rep career had been on hold ever since her prize recruit, Dr. Luke Cameron, went rogue and had to be dealt with publicly. His failure had reflected badly on her. It was a huge blot on her record and came with a painful cut in pay.

Jen reluctantly opened the stupid file she'd been handed. It was a standard request for information regarding any public drug testing conducted by Global Pharm. The reason for the request mentioned a patient with unusual blue irises. Jen wasn't sure why, but Dr. Luke Cameron came to mind when she read about the blue irises.

He'd received a Code Nine dismissal. Talk about harsh punishment. He'd never work in the Pharmaceutical industry again, and for what? For curing a rat of something or other she recalled. She'd only caught a glimpse of Cameron's file when her former Rep Manager had slammed it down on his desk while reprimanding her. The pages had spilled out in front of her and she'd read what she could while her boss ranted on about how critical recruiting standards were. She hadn't been able to read the entire file, but whatever Cameron had discovered it had pissed off the Board and it had side effects, one to be exact.

On the closest page spread out in front of her, Jen remembered seeing a report stating ...one side effect... startling blue irises. She'd read that just seconds before her Manager demoted her and had her removed bodily from his office.

It was a long shot, but if that damned Luke Cameron was trying to recreate the Cure with the same side effect then the patient from this file could be part of his experiment. A surge of adrenaline flushed her cheeks.

She had to be sure, but if it was Cameron, she'd track him down and end his folly. She'd drag his ass back to Global Pharm with proof of his illegal and unethical experiments on humans. That would end the threat of another Cure, bring her back into the good graces of the Industry and get her out of this hell hole of a job she'd been banished to.

Jen still held the title of Rep, despite her demotion. She took advantage of her Superior being on holidays and used her "Rep" clout to requisition a plane ticket and corporate SUV for a drug recall field investigation. She desperately needed to question the patient with the blue irises while he was still in the hospital. She cleared her desk, hopefully for the last time, raced home and packed an overnight bag then headed for the airport.

Her flight arrived the very next day. It took her less than an hour to exit the airport, hail a taxi and check in at the local field office. She picked up her black Global Pharm SUV and drove straight to the hospital, skipping breakfast. While dodging morning traffic she used the on board computer, linked to amongst other things, the e-health data base. Jen knew what room her prey was in before she parked.

She took all the steps she'd been taught as a Rep to remain unseen by hospital staff. Upon entering his room, Jen quietly pulled back the curtain surrounding his bed.

Rob Burnett looked up angrily from the latest swimsuit edition of Sports Illustrated he'd been enjoying. When he saw the blonde knock out standing at the foot of his bed, he sat up and smiled.

Jen smiled back using her sexiest smile and pulled the curtain closed behind her. "Hello Mr. Burnett, my name's Jen Hanson." She used her sexy *you're cute* voice on him, stepping forward to shake his hand. "I'm a Rep from Global Pharm. How do you feel? Are you in any pain?"

Rob was flustered by this sexy beauty alone behind the curtain with him. He was so excited he'd already forgotten her name. He took her warm outstretched hand saying, "My head hurts."

"Oh dear," she fretted, "That's one of the side effects I'm afraid." Jen paused for dramatic effect. She wanted this guy worried, curious and compliant before starting her interrogation.

"But don't fret, if we can figure out exactly what was done to you, we can probably reverse it. Trust me."

"Why? What's been done to me?!" Rob asked in terror.

Good, thought Jan and got down to work. "I'm so sorry to be the one to tell you Mr. Burnett, you may have been exposed to a potentially deadly drug. It was created in our labs without our knowledge, by a deeply troubled former employee. Now he's running around experimenting on innocent people like you."

"Who? Dr. Cameron?!" Rob interjected.

"That's right, Dr. Cameron, poor man. He tried some of the drug on himself and well, it has more than just one side effect. Only after it was too late did our best researchers discover that the drug also corrupts the mind, eventually leading to madness. Blue irises are the first danger sign, then the headaches."

Rob's eyes widened a bit as fear ran an icy finger up his spine. "I knew there was something odd about that guy. It sounded too good to be true. He said it would cure my Diabetes," he said and Jen detected a touch of embarrassment in his voice.

"Cure Diabetes?" she laughed, "We're still a number of years away from that I'm afraid," lied Jen aloud, but to herself she thought, "Christ! this is bigger than I'd imagined."

"So what's gonna happen to me? I don't want to go nuts, and my head *really* hurts now" said Rob trying to hide his panic.

"Well you're in luck Rob. May I call you Rob?" he nodded excitedly. "Thanks," she continued, "Our researchers have been able to develop a counter agent to Dr. Cameron's drug. I have it right here," she cooed, withdrawing from her purse a standard issue neuro toxin filled syringe.

This wouldn't be her first cover up murder, but before finishing the job she asked Rob if there was anything else he could tell her. She sat beside him near the intravenous stand.

Completely unaware of the mortal danger he was in Rob split open like a ripe melon and told her everything. He was scared and embarrassed. He wanted Cameron caught and punished for what he'd done. He'd tricked him, giving him real hope with a fake cure. Well he wasn't going to get away with it. Rob saw the only way he could get the last laugh, and he began talking.

When Rob had told her as much as he knew and started repeating himself, Jen stood up. "Thank you Mr. Burnett, you've been most helpful." Then she calmly uncapped the needle Rob took to be the counter agent.

She inserted the needle into his I.V. tube, depressing the plunger. Rob's smile showed his relief. "There you go sweetie, soon you won't have anything to worry about," whispered Jen into his ear. By the time she finished Rob Burnett was staring blankly at the ceiling, dead. No longer living proof of a cure.

Now all Jen had to do was find Dr. Cameron. According to Rob, he'd been cured almost a week ago in a small town just a couple of hours drive North of the Hospital.

Jen left Rob's room unobserved, exactly as she'd entered it. Then grabbed a bite to eat and drove straight to the small town. She figured on being there late afternoon depending on traffic.

Luke rode his bike out of town Wednesday morning on schedule. Right after making the necessary follow up house calls to all his Chosen patients, except Mr Burnett. Luke had stopped by as arranged, but no-one had answered when he'd knocked on the door. He hadn't waited long either. He hadn't liked Mr. Burnett that much anyway. Ms. Green had turned out to be his thousandth cured Diabetic.

The follow up appointment was the deal sealer. If the Chosen hadn't given in to temptation and become Diabetics again, he gave them a second injection. It was that second dose that made their Cure permanent. Luke had learned that after Mark's relapse and subsequent second dose. So he'd separated the Cure into two doses given up to a week apart. Any longer than that, the cure broke down, became undetectable and the person's Diabetes returned. It was his final test.

Luke had loaded the payments collected from the Chosen into his bike's carrier. When that was full he used the saddlebags. Any more weight and he'd have had trouble keeping the front wheel on the ground. As it was he had to lean forward while he rode.

Fifty kilometers from the small town Dr. Cameron pulled into a quiet little trailer park off the main road. He stopped in at the office, then rode down the main trail until he saw Chloe and the kids sitting in front of their Winnebago. The one L.J. had given them three years ago as payment for his cure. Their touring bikes were courtesy of Olga.

"Hi everyone, are we ready to go?" Luke asked, trying to stay on schedule.

"We thought we'd have lunch first then go. Is there any rush?" asked Chloe as she flipped the juicy hamburgers on the grill.

"Nope, not that I'm aware of," said Luke brushing back his hair again. He unloaded his bike's carrier, assigning Fran to help store the gifts, his bag and bike this time. Once that was done he sat down to eat and tell them what the Chosen had been like in this town.

"Oh I cured my thousanth Diabetic," boasted Luke. They all applauded until he got up and took a bow. It was probably the only recognition he'd ever receive, but he was receiving it from the people he loved and respected the most.

Later that afternoon as they were travelling down the road they passed a black SUV heading in the opposite direction. Luke was the only one to recognize the Global Pharm logo on its front doors. He couldn't help but notice the attractive blonde driving.

In a blinding flash he realized who it was, and who he hoped it wasn't… Jen Hanson, the Rep from hell.

He checked the rear view mirror to make sure she hadn't recognized him. Then he remembered he was in disguise and thanked his lucky stars. The SUV continued towards the town Luke had just left. That was too close, he needed a minute to think. *What was a Rep doing way out here? Could it be about me? Naw, couldn't be, we've been so careful. It's gotta be a coincidence, but if not…?*

He pulled over at a rest stop and brushed his annoying shock of auburn hair from his forehead again. Then without warning he bellowed, "That's it!" and grabbing the infuriating hair with his fist, ripped it from his head.

"Man that was the wig from hell! Do me a favor Chloe, no more wigs, just dye my hair again for the next town, Okay?" begged Luke taking off his glasses, tossing them on the dash and rubbing his bald head vigorously.

The whole family slowly took off their disguises and relaxed. Over the years, the Chosen had picked a wide variety of methods to pay for their cures.

One of the first payments had come from Udo the makeup artist and town hairstylist. He'd given them a dozen wigs, colored contact lenses, makeup and a crash course on applying everything.

Another had worked at the government passport office and created several false passports for each of them. Another had produced fake driver's licenses. Most recently Mrs. Roberta Green had given Luke $100,000 in tens and twenties, saying it was all she could scrape together to aid his crusade.

All in all, it was a good life. The family enjoyed travelling, and the work was rewarding. They just had to stay one step ahead of the drug companies.

So far that hadn't been a problem, but seeing Jen Hanson that close again had sent a chill up Luke's spine. He suddenly felt the need to get as far away from there as possible.

Not wanting to alarm anyone, Luke reached over to take the well-used road map from the glove box and opened it up. "Well boys and girls, where should we make our next house call?"

Chapter 5
Strange Reactions

I was once given a book that saved my life and started a chain reaction of events that took me from Huntsville Canada to New York City, where I saved the life of the book's Author. True Story.

It all started one snowy morning, days before Christmas 2009. I'd taken a Taxi ride to a medical appointment in Huntsville, but couldn't get a Taxi back. Undeterred, I started walking/hitch-hiking home. I've always enjoyed a good stretch of the legs, but then it started snowing lightly. "What next?" I sighed, tempting fate and sticking out my thumb at the sound of an approaching vehicle. A silver van pulled over just ahead of me and stopped.

I'd barely climbed in, when the driver asked, "So how'd you like that party the other night?"

"?"…Swear to God, I had no idea who this guy was.

"Don't you recognize me?" he asked gruffly. I turned for a better look. He was fiftyish, thinning brown hair, moustache, wore a tan parka, glasses and an expectant smile. Finally, with an exasperated sigh he said, "I'm your Optometrist…" then paused, as if that was enough of a clue for anyone to finish the sentence. I was still drawing blanks. "…Jim?" he finished.

"Guess I need new glasses, eh doc?" I joked.

Jim frowned. "You've got Diabetes, right?" "Yeah…" I admitted warily, expecting a lecture about Diabetes retinopathy or something

"Me too, just got it," he confided, surprising me. "I'm not taking the pills though. I'll control my blood sugars with diet and exercise instead," he quickly added.

I've heard that before...never seen it work. "Good luck with that," I encouraged skeptically. "I've been taking needles for forty seven years, myself."

Jim naturally started picking my brain about Diabetes. He grew increasingly concerned as he heard the lifestyle requirements he'd need to adopt. All his Diabetic patients had complications and he feared the same fate.

"Living with Diabetes is hard at first," I agreed. "It's mostly trial & error. Errors cause complications if you don't correct them. Too bad there's no guide book."

Ironically, Jim *had* found a guidebook of sorts on the internet: "Diabetes Solutions." "It's written by a Doctor who's had Diabetes for sixty four years!" I raised an impressed eyebrow. "I've ordered copies to give to my Diabetic patients."

Arriving out front of my house, Jim parked the van and began rummaging through the grey duffle bag between our seats. "You read, right?" he asked, hauling out a dauntingly thick hardcover book. "Here," he grunted as he tossed it to me, adding a curt, "Merry Christmas."

The author was Dr. Richard Bernstein. "Bernstein? He's not that diet guy is he?" I asked disdainfully. "Nope," reassured Jim. So I gratefully accepted his unexpected gift. We shook hands, I wished him a Merry Christmas, opened the door, climbed out and headed for my front door, full of questions.

Why had I ended up with this book? It hadn't been intended for me. Should I read the book? Was I meant to read the book? Of course, why else would I have it. Would it, could it, help me?

I read that book during the holidays, cover to cover. It was inspiring. On January first, 2010, my wife Susan and I made some simple changes to our daily routine.

The results were dramatic & surprising. From the very first day, I easily kept my sugars between 4.0 & 7.0. Funny, I'd hated testing before. Seeing nothing but highs & lows was depressing. Guilt & frustration had plagued me.

Now, I actually *anticipated* testing. It became a game, how many results in the 4-7 range could I get in a row? (Seven). I was in control!!!

I began to promote Bernstein's book. Susan bought a dozen copies and I gave one to every Diabetic I knew or met.

Bernstein became my Diabetic hero.

In February, I suffered a setback. Despite near perfect blood sugars, I lost a long battle with an infection and a second toe was amputated. Undaunted, I continued regulating my sugars and healed way faster than usual.

One March morning, while we were getting dressed, Susan paused and looked me up & down. "You've lost weight," she cooed approvingly. "Look who's talking," I replied, nodding towards the mirror. Without effort, we'd lost 10 kilos each. Fantastic.

April, I went to what was only my 2nd eye exam with Jim. I brought line graphs, created using my test results, to demonstrate the difference Bernstein's book had made. Jim was impressed with my success, confessing that he hadn't read the book himself. He also admitted to taking pills for his Diabetes now.

A week later Jim sent me an e-mailed that read,

"Attending the Metabolism and Nutrition Society's meeting in New York May seventh. Have an extra plane ticket. Guest speaker is Dr. Bernstein. Want to go?"

How cool is that?! These unexpected opportunities are the spice in my life.

My reply was a simple, "Yes." Maybe I'd get Bernstein's autograph.

First evening in New York, we joined other M & NS members for dinner at an outdoor restaurant with a great view of the Statue of Liberty. Everyone at our table was a Doctor with a degree and published book. Everyone except me.

I'm just a high school graduate with a handful of graph paper. Plus Jim and I were the only Diabetics there. Many people there knew each other from previous meetings and held conversations regarding absent colleagues. Talk about feeling out of place and alienated. Over the course of the evening I kept asking myself, *Why am I here?*

Next morning we headed out for breakfast before the meeting. Exiting our Hotel, we were instantly swept into the torrent of pedestrians flowing by. Every time Jim was cut off, shoved or blocked, he'd shout, "This is insane!" to me over the calliope of downtown sounds. I just smiled and minded my wallet. We navigated our way, bumping and cursing, to a diner. Then cursed and bumped to the meeting.

The meeting was held in a lecture room on the fourth floor of a posh nearby Hotel. Inside the room were several rows of tables and chairs. To my left was a door to an adjoining room with a buffet & refreshments. To my right was a raised platform with projection screen. The room was already half full with people reading their orientation packages, or talking quietly. I took a seat on the far side of the room by the wall of windows.

The meeting started with the hostess announcing "Dr. Bernstein is running late." Another lecturer was called upon to speak until he arrived. Twenty minutes later my hero entered the room.

I don't know what I'd been expecting Bernstein to look like, but it sure wasn't this frail, little old man. He was trembling as he was led by the arm to the raised platform. He appeared anxious. When the hostess let go of him, he teetered unsteadily, threatening to fall. She caught him just in time and a volunteer brought him a chair.

When he spoke, his words were slurred & confused, fading in and out. *Is he having a stroke?* I wondered. He bowed his head and drifted into a momentary silence. Abruptly he sat up, shook his head and tried vainly to continue.

Obviously, something was wrong with him. Something oddly familiar. In a flash of insight, I understood. He was having a 'Reaction'! Sugars so low they can kill a Diabetic!

"He needs sugar," I prompted, loud enough for the Doctors and Nurses around me to hear. A half roll of life-savers was slowly passed forward. I knew from experience that wasn't nearly enough sugar.

I grabbed my kit. I carry it with me most of the time. It's got a meter, test strips, lancets, two pen needles and a tube of Dextrose (sugar tablets). The life-savers hadn't reached Dr. Bernstein before he collapsed into the waiting arms of the hostess. He was helped to a seat at a nearby table.

The room fell silent.

Nobody moved.

I couldn't believe it. Shouldn't this room full of Doctors be falling all over each other to save this guy? Apparently, no-one else realized what was happening, or how deadly serious it was. I stood up. Diabetics have to watch out for one another.

Quickly crossing the room, I crouched beside Dr. Bernstein. He appeared unconscious, slumped over the table, head resting on his folded arms, eyes closed. I touched his arm, cold and clammy, a bad sign. If his sugars dropped too low, he'd slip into a coma!

"Dr. Bernstein, I'm a Diabetic. I'm going to test your blood sugars," I explained calmly. He was silent. I pricked his finger and had to squeeze his finger a few times before I got the drop of blood for the test. Another bad sign.

A Doctor and Nurse came to watch what I was doing. "He's 1.8," I advised them, grabbing the tube of Dextrose from my kit. He needed sugar immediately or he'd die before an ambulance could arrive.

"What's 1.8 in American?" asked the Nurse. They use a different scale to measure blood sugars in the States. "Multiply by eighteen," I recalled from Bernstein's book while shaking tablets from the tube. Talk about irony.

"That's only thirty four," exclaimed the Doctor.

"Oh my," gasped the Nurse, realizing the danger.

I placed a comforting hand on Dr. Bernstein's back, and tried to slip a dextrose tablet past his lips. He started shaking & convulsing. When I did finally manage to get a Dextrose tablet into his mouth, he spat it out.

Come on Doc this is no time to be picky, I thought, pushing the tablet back in and helping him sip some water to dissolve it quicker.

"Want some Orange juice?" the Nurse interrupted politely.

"Please," I urged, kicking myself for not thinking of it first.

After the fourth Dextrose tablet, Dr. Bernstein stopped shaking. The hostess came over and asked if we could get him out of the room, he was distracting the other members. We moved him to a chair in the hallway, where he produced a tube of *liquid* dextrose from his briefcase and sucked it dry. Then he shut his eyes, hung his head and waited to feel normal again. Been there, done that.

Five tense minutes later when he finally raised his head and opened his eyes, I was the first person he saw. "Who are you?" I introduced myself.

"Boy, they grow em big in Canada, don't they?" he teased. The Doctor, Nurse, hostess and I all chuckled with relief. He looked me right in the eye and said, "Thanks". He didn't have to say, "for saving his life." I could see it in his weary eyes.

A rapturous joy swelled in my chest, filling it to bursting. I'd saved a life, my Diabetic hero's life. I inhaled deeply to calm myself. "You're welcome," I replied coolly. "Can I have your autograph?"

Chapter 6
Whirlpool

It was the middle of summer vacation for Robby, his brother Steven and little sister Wendy. They were lying around the house, bored.

"What do you want to do?" Robby asked Steven.

"I don't know," answered Steven uncaringly.

"What do you want to do?" Steven asked Wendy, slowly rolling his eyes towards her. She was laying upside down in her Mom's favorite chair, staring blankly at the TV.

"Ohh, I don't know, what do you guys want to do?"

"Why don't you go out and play?" suggested their Mom.

"Aw Mom, it's way too hot to play outside," the kids protested together.

"Even if we went for a swim?" asked their Mom with an encouraging smile. Robby sat up quickly, but trying to sound cool said, "All right."

Steven yelled, "All right!" jumping up off the couch and bolting to his room to get his new swimming trunks on. Six year old Wendy said, "Okay," with a nervous waver in her voice. After all, she'd only had a couple of swimming lessons.

Their pool was a big oval above ground, twenty four feet long, eighteen wide and four and a half deep, perfect for children. Their Dad had it built so only a foot was above ground with one step up onto the surrounding eight foot wide brown cedar deck.

"Can we invite friends?" the three of them begged their Mom.

"Sure, sure, just not every kid on the street," she cautioned. So Robby called Teddy and Willy who lived next door Steven called Evan, and his brother Kevin.

Wendy asked Mom to call her bestest friends; Betty, and the identical twins Jenny & Penny.
Everyone they invited shouted "Yeah!"

Robby ran to the fridge and drank some Orange juice. He was Diabetic and knew that he needed extra energy for swimming or he'd have a reaction. He hated reactions. They made him weak and confused.

One minute later the doorbell rang. Mom opened the front door and saw a gaggle of excited children waiting outside. They all wore bathing suits, flip-flops & sunglasses except Willy. He was wearing a cool scuba mask.

Everyone brought a beach towel. They were colorful, bright and festive. All except Kevin's, he had a thick white bath towel with, "Property of Motel 6," stenciled across it in big black letters.

The boys had their towels slung over a shoulder, trying not to appear too excited or foolish in front of the girls. They were pushing and shoving each other playfully to release their pent up energy.

The girls had their towels wrapped around their waists like Polynesian skirts. They each wore a different colored bathing cap. Betty's was hot pink with white flowers along the edges. They were huddled together, sneaking peeks at the bare chested boys, then whispering to each other and giggling.

Mom knew the kids would push past her any second and tear through her freshly cleaned house if she didn't act quick.

"Okay everyone, go around to the backyard and I'll go unlock the gate," she said, pointing right. The excited mob of kids stampeded around the house for the backyard.

"Last one in's a rotten egg," yelled Kenny as they rounded the last corner and saw the pool.

Every kid started pumping their legs faster, screaming and yelling as they pushed, shoved and cajoled each other.

They had trouble stopping and piled into each other at the locked pool gate. Mom opened the back door, releasing Robby, Steven and Wendy. They ran over to the pool gate and joined their panting friends. Mom excused her way through the chest high crowd, unlocked the gate and opened it, unleashing all nine kids.

They gushed through the narrow gate, carelessly tossing their colorful towels into the air and cascading into the pool, churning the water into a frothy foam that spread across the surface.

Little Wendy didn't dive into the pool with the others. She had to wear a blow up plastic ring to stay afloat. She wore it around her waist when she jumped in, but when she came up sputtering, it was up under her arms. She dug her fingers into it and hanging on for dear life, kicked and bobbed her way towards the security of the pool edge.

Mom hadn't had time to fish out the floating chlorine basket before the kids went in. After frolicking and splashing each other for several minutes, Teddy complained.

"My eyes are burning," he cried rubbing his eyes with the heel of his hands.

"That's how come I got a mask," boasted Kevin.

"Not any more," corrected Steven, snatching the mask off Kevin's head. Steven half ran, half swam away, holding the mask just out of Kevin's reach.

"Hey! Come on give em back, they're my Dad's," yelled Kevin running & hopping through the water in a vain attempt to catch Steven.

The two boys raced through the water following the curved edge of the pool. Round and round they went, Steven running backwards to torment poor Kevin.

Soon they had created a swirling current in the pool, and a strong one at that. The floating toys Mom had been tossing in for the kids were gathering in the center of the pool.

"Hey look at the bottom of the pool," said Penny. "All the sand is collecting in the middle."

Sure enough, Steven and Kevin were creating a whirlpool. Some children tried to cling to the side of the pool so as not to be swept away.

"Let's all run along the side and see how strong we can make it" suggested Willy.

All the boys all yelled "Yeah," let go of the pool edge and ran with the current.

The girls all looked nervous. They were already having trouble hanging onto the pool edge. The boys started running as fast as they could through the water, in one direction.

The girls pulled themselves along the edge of the pool cautiously, scared to let go. Fearful that if they let go they might never get out.

Robby, the biggest boy, turned and planted his feet on the pool bottom in defiance of the current. It pushed him over and dragged him under in a heartbeat. Popping up a second later he joined the others as they ran on chanting "fas-ter, fas-ter, fas-ter!"

Mom had been sitting in a deck chair sunning when the commotion started. She cast a weary glance towards the pool.

"Okay that's enough, stop running around like that Wendy can't hang on." True enough, but no-one could.

In fact, the current was now so strong that getting out was a problem. The ladder had been pushed on it's side by the rushing water so no one could climb out. Robby could barely hold on to the side of the pool, and every time he jumped up to get out, his legs were forced sideways and he plunged back in.

The younger kids, with their blow up rings, were bobbing along the edge of the pool like corks caught in a wild river.

Everyone was tuckered out from making the whirlpool, fighting against it, and all the failed attempts at escaping it. Robby finally managed to haul himself onto the deck by jumping up and grabbing the diving board as he passed under it.

He lay on the deck on his back, gasping, his heart hammering in his chest. Then he heard the other kids calling for help. He turned his head to see his mom chasing after them as they went whipping around the pool edge. *That is one wicked whirlpool,* he thought.

Wendy came racing towards him. "Grab my hand Robby I want to get out," whined Wendy choking and sputtering. Robby could tell she was about to burst into tears. She was bobbing up and down, but managed to raise one desperate hand while clutching the ring with the other.

Robby couldn't roll over fast enough to reach her outstretched hand as she flashed past.
Oops, man she's really moving, realized Robby as he struggled to his knees. The next kid approaching was just a pair of feet. It had to be Steven, he was the only kid around who could walk on his hands.

Robby knew he had to act fast to get a grip on Steven's ankles as he sped by, but he hesitated. *What if I can't get his head out of the water and he drowns? Mom & Dad would be pretty mad at me for a while.*

There was no time to worry about it. Robby grabbed his brother's ankles and pulled with all his remaining strength. Steven came out of the water, arms flailing, eyes shut, and landed on his back with a smack.

Robby, Steven their Mom started hauling the kids out as quick as they could catch hold of them. Five exhausting minutes later, all the kids were safely out,

Mom flopped back into her sunning chair. The kids lay around the pool on their backs, gasping like a school of fish out of water.

Wendy sat up first. Her inflatable ring hung limply around her waist. She'd been clutching it so tight she'd punctured it. Mom looked over at her and shook her head, sure that Wendy would never go swimming again after this. But Wendy rubbed her burning eyes and said, "That was fun. Let's do it again?"

Chapter 7
First Jump

Looking around my writing room, searching for something to trigger my next story, I spotted an old blue and white certificate. It was hanging on the wall amongst other treasured mementos from my wilder days. A smile spread across my face, and I feel the twinkle in my eye grow brighter as I recall the first time I went parachuting.

It was back in 1980. I'd opened my first business, a landscaping company, employing eight full time and six part time people, mostly friends and family. We did everything from home yard maintenance, to office and apartment building grounds maintenance. From flower planting, weeding and fertilizing, to tree planting and pruning. I worked seven days a week for months on end, only taking a day off if it rained.

On one of those drizzly overcast mornings in late September, about an hour after I'd sent my crew home, I got a strange phone call from one of them, Pete Detwiler. We'd been friends for years and he'd jumped at the chance to work with me. I liked Pete, he was a good worker, had a great sense of humor and shared a kindred spirit of adventure.

"Whatcha doin?" his tone told me he didn't give a rats ass what I was doing, he had something better.
"Catch'n up on some paperwork, why? What's up?"
"Ughhh paperwork, sounds boring. Want to go skydiving instead?"

"Skydiving!?" I asked dubiously, but quickly added, "Where?"
"You know where Arthur is eh?" he asked.

"Nope," I replied. We lived in Mississauga at the time, and although I'd travelled to Europe, Mexico and Hawaii, I hadn't travelled much through rural Ontario.

"Well it's about an hour North of here, I'll even drive. Whudaya say, wanna go?" he prodded.

"How much," I asked, figuring it'd be hundreds of dollars, a good enough excuse to say no.

"Nintey nine bucks," he said enthusiastically.

"That's all?" I said surprised, and started to feel that old familiar sense of adventure kick in.

"Yup, I read the ad in this morning's paper and called them. We take indoor classes all morning, write a test, train all afternoon and jump at the end of the day," he elaborated, and I could hear the, "What's the problem? Let's go already," in his voice.

We were both silent for a moment, him waiting and me thinking. Parachuting *was* one of those things I'd always wanted to do, but never had the opportunity before. I was twenty one, invincible, immortal, owner of a successful business, why not throw myself from a plane?

I looked at my watch. It was already 9:00 am. "What time do the classes start?" I asked.

"Nine," said Pete, "We gotta go right now. I'll be over in five minutes to pick you up. Meet me downstairs in the lobby, Okay?"

"Perfect," I said hanging up. I made a PB & J sandwich, wrapped it up and threw some carrot sticks into a baggie. Then grabbed a couple of packs of raisins in case of low blood sugars, (There were no dextrose tablets back then), and shoved them all into a paper bag.

I put an extra pack of smokes and some sugar packets (also in case of low sugars) into my shirt's breast pocket. In 1980, Diabetics didn't have Glucometers to check their blood sugar levels.

Controlling my Diabetes was all about taking my needle at the same time every day, getting some exercise and sticking to my diet. The only variable was the amount of exercise I got. Too much and my blood sugars dropped causing a life threatening 'Reaction'.

I hate Reactions they feel like a slice of death. To recover from a Reaction, all I used to do was eat or drink something sweet. A few minutes later, I'd be right as rain, but soaked in sweat. That reminded me to pack an extra T-shirt just in case.

I'd had Diabetes for about 17 years by this point in my life. I knew what to expect from most day to day happenings, but Parachuting would be something completely different. I've always looked forward to any new experience that expands my knowledge of Diabetes care and control.

Pete was waiting in his black Mustang when I got downstairs. We drove to Arthur singing along and playing air guitar to the assorted Rock and Roll cassette tapes he had. When we got to Arthur we found the airfield was in the middle of a farmer's field.

There was a barn, a farm house and a cedar post & wire fence running off into a distant stand of trees. The runway ran straight down the middle of a hundred acre field and ended between the barn and the forest. A great big three ring target was painted at that end of the runway. Fifty yards past the target was a row of yellow school busses parked in front of the wire fence separating the airfield from the farmer's field next door.

"Thiz muzt be da plaze," I joked as Pete drove down the long gravel driveway. We parked in front of the farm house, at the far end of a long line of cars.

Inside the old house, a class of about forty people were going on break, squeezing by us as we stuck our heads in the doorway. "Al" the instructor strode over to Pete and I and shook our hands vigorously. "Glad you could make it, Dan, Paul," he said taking a poor stab at our names. "Dave and Pete,'" I corrected, but he just kept smiling and handed us clipboards with registration forms. "Have a seat boys," he said, pointing to a couple of seats at the front of the room.

While filling out the forms and signing the multiple waivers, Al explained that because we were late, we'd have to miss lunch. That was so we could watch the film and take the test everyone else had just finished. Pete said, "No problem," but I *had* to have a lunch, it was part of my daily routine. Good thing I'd brought my own.

After signing up and paying Al, we joined the others. They came from all over: Toronto, Hamilton, Guelph and Kitchener to name a few. There was a good mixture of men and women with a surprisingly wide range of ages, from sixteen to sixty.

The sixty year old, Marge, was bursting with excited smiles. She said, "Oh Boy," when we were introduced to the rest of the class. Later I found out she was only there because her granddaughter, Judy, had bought tickets for both of them as Marge's sixtieth birthday present. As long as Judy was jumping too, Marge figured, "Why not?"

The rest of the morning was full of cool information. Al reminded us that the best scientific minds in the world could not devise a better, or safer, method to return space capsules to Earth than the parachute.

"You'll be using the WW II Dome parachutes. The ones that look like a giant mushroom cap." Later we found out that the modern rectangular chutes, which Al and the other experienced jumpers used, were highly maneuverable, used in professional competitions and very expensive.

"You'll be jumping from twenty eight hundred feet, a thousand feet higher than the CN Tower. If your main chute doesn't open, it'll only take you thirteen seconds to plummet to the ground." The entire class gasped as one, sucking all the air from the room.

"If your main chute doesn't open, there *is* an emergency chute on the front of your parachute harness. You have to throw your emergency chute out by hand," he continued as if that bit of news would reassure us.

Marge said, "Oh boy," which sounded like, "Oh no," to me. I counted to thirteen in my head. It didn't feel like enough time to realize something was wrong and remember what to do about it while tumbling through the air at close to two hundred miles per hour. Color me slow.

During the lunch break, everyone went to eat at a local restaurant in town, except us. I gave Pete half my sandwich and we ate to the whir of the reel to reel film about parachutes. Then we wrote the test, passing with flying colors.

After lunch, the group returned to the classroom. Pete leaned over and whispered,"Looks like we lost a few." Sure enough, when I counted heads, at least four people were missing from this morning's class.

Al stuck his head in the door and said, "Okay, now the fun really starts. Come on." Marge said, "Oh Boy," but sounded a bit nervous.

With Al in the lead, we all trooped from the nice warm house out into the windy, drizzle filled, cold. We raced across the thirty yards to the red and white barn with the grey metal roof.

Inside, the barn was one big open space. I could see from front to back and all the way up to the rafters some forty feet above our heads. Off in the corner to our left, were two guys hunched over a long wooden bench. They were folding and packing nylon chutes into square canvas back packs.

"Are we going to learn how to fold our chutes?" asked the youngest member of the class, a sixteen year old blonde girl there with her father. I never got their names.

"No, but I like your enthusiasm," chuckled Al. "Only trained and certified "Riggers" are allowed to pack chutes. Right now, you're going to learn to jump and land on that big pillow over there," he said pointing to a twenty foot square, four foot deep mesh bag, loosely stuffed with coarse, head sized chunks of soft brown foam rubber.

"Oh boy," said Marge, sounding more nervous than ever. "Don't be afraid, go check it out," insisted Al. Some people put their hands on it and leaned in to see how much give there was. Others threw themselves on top of it to see what it felt like. Laughter and dust particles quickly filled the air, mingling with the nervous excitement already there.

"Okay, that's enough, half of you up the ladder, the other half spread out around the foam pillow," instructed Al. He was standing at the foot of a hand-made wooden ladder that led up to a platform 20 ft. above us. It stretched from one side of the barn to the other.

Pete and I were the first two up the ladder. There was a single bare sixty watt bulb burning way above our heads. It gave just enough light to see that there was nothing up there on that eight foot wide platform but us. The roughhewn planks underfoot were slightly uneven and one sagged a bit and creaked when I stepped on it.

Fifteen of us lined up along the platform's rounded edge and cautiously stuck our heads over to see where the bag of foam was. It was directly under me, but looked a lot smaller from up here. It reminded me of the Bugs Bunny cartoon where Bugs is about to dive from a ridiculously high platform into a bucket of water, and pulls out a pair of binoculars so he can see the bucket and take aim.

"Okay, first person step forward," said Al calling up to us from beside the pillow. I stepped up to the edge dead center of the pillow below.

"Remember to bend your knees and roll to the side when you land, okay?"

I just nodded and gave him the thumbs up. I'm always nervous about being the example for others to either follow or avoid. I hesitated just long enough to remember how much I hated people who lost their nerve at the last moment. They'd stand there, searching vainly for the courage they'd had just a moment ago, holding up the line and frustrating everyone.

I bent my knees and jumped just high and far enough to clear the edge of the platform. I counted to two before feeling the soft uneven foam under my feet. I sank into the pillow, quickly hitting bottom and rolling to the right.

I'd landed dead center and almost rolled off, but helping hands guided me off the pillow and onto my feet in one smooth move.

"Good one," said Al, "Next."

Pete was next, then 60 year old Marge, who said, "Oh Boy," a couple of times, before she jumped. And a couple more times after rolling off the foam with a big smile lighting up her face.

When everyone up on the platform had jumped, Al sent the other half of the class up and we got to "Spot" them as they jumped.

The fourth person, a short fat bald man, had trouble jumping. His eyes darted from the foam pillow to the rafters several times. He held up the line for a second until we all started chanting, "Jump, Jump, Jump...," louder and louder. We weren't being mean, we were encouraging him.

Finally, with a final glance up, he closed his eyes took a deep breath and jumped. The little guy landed on his ass and hit hard enough that we heard it.

He sat there for a moment, shocked and embarrassed. We all started applauding and cheering. He smiled back, rolling onto his belly and crawling across the netting to the edge of the pillow. He was helped off by his red faced wife and two proud adolescent children.

Once we'd all jumped, Al made us repeat the exercise. Pete and I were first up the ladder again. This time he jumped first.

After we'd all jumped a few times Al led the group to a contraption that looked like a child's swing set made of four by four posts. It stood ten feet tall at the crossbar and the side braces were eight feet apart. There were three braces on each side making it look very sturdy.

"Now we're going to strap you into the parachute harness, hang you up from the cross bar here and show you how to deploy your emergency chute. Remember, 1 in 1000 main chutes malfunctions." The group fell silent as the statistic sank in and everyone asked themselves, "Am I that one in a thousand?"

"Oh come on, only one in a hundred and eighty thousand malfunctions are fatal," he added quickly to reassure us. Pete and I looked at each other and shrugged. We were both twenty one years old, and virtually indestructible. The worst thing that would happen if our chutes didn't open was we'd bounce more than three times when we hit the ground.

"Alright then, who wants to be our airline stewardess and demonstrate how to put on the parachute harness?" asked Al as two Riggers came over with armfuls of harnesses.

We each took one and watched as Marge was strapped in and cinched tight. She squealed "Oh Boy," in a high-pitched voice when they tightened the two crotch straps.

Once we were all strapped in, Al told us to line up in front of one of the four wooden contraptions. Under each crossbar was a three rung step ladder. The first person in each line, which included me, climbed the steps. The Riggers clipped our harness' shoulder rings to wire cables hanging from the cross bar.

Our straps were given a final tightening, almost castrating me, except for my instinctive hip swivel. Nonetheless, when the stepladder was removed, my entire one hundred and eighty pounds, was carried by the straps between my legs. It was an awkward and uncomfortable position to be in.

Two wooden handles hung from bungie chords attached to the cross bar. They represented our steering toggles. We learned to steer our chute by pulling on these toggles which open flaps on the chute called Rills. The toggles automatically drop down when the chute opens.

The square satchel, containing the emergency chute was attached to the straps of my harness right where they crossed my chest.

"Okay, now listen up," said Al and I hoped he was going to be brief.

"If you have to manually deploy your emergency chute, pull this chord," he pointed to the red toggled chord. "That opens the pack on your chest. Then you reach into the pack, putting one hand, palm out, under the chute and the other hand on top of the chute and throw it outwards like this."

Oh it sounded easy enough, but when you're suspended mid-air, any movement causes you to wobble on the cables, throwing off your balance. When I pulled the chord, I wobbled wildly and had to keep kicking my legs to keep from flipping over.

Getting as close to upright as possible, I grabbed the chute the way I'd been shown and tossed it way out in front of me. I threw it so hard it almost completely unfurled, chords and all.

It took a while, but we all tried the emergency chute throwing at least once. Then Al called a well deserved coffee break and the class split up. I grabbed a coffee while Pete went to take a leak.

When our class got back together, fifteen minutes later, even fewer people had returned. I counted them, only thirty left now. Al didn't mention the missing people and neither did we. Fortune favors the bold.

Al took us back outside for a little landing practice. The drizzle had stopped, but the low hanging clouds were an ominous dark grey. A strong wind was still blowing out of the west, making the airfield's wind sock stand straight out.

"If the weather keeps up like this we may have to postpone the jump," warned Al looking up at the sky's dark grey belly.

Al led us to the far side of the barn, thankfully out of the wind. There was a small wooden platform there, about six feet high and four wide, with uneven wooden stairs. Marge's granddaughter, a cute sixteen year old blonde was the first to climb the stairs.

"Right, now step up to the far edge. When you jump down from there, land on your toes, with your knees bent and angled to one side, roll to that side, when you land," said Al.

"Another important thing to remember on the way down is never look at the ground between your feet. Your senses will be distorted when you land and a blade of grass can look as big as a tree if you're looking down. Safer to look at the horizon when you land then your legs will absorb the impact." With a nod from Al,

Marge's granddaughter jumped down and rolled to the side perfectly, setting the benchmark for the rest of us.

When it was my turn I stepped up to the edge and was surprised how high six feet actually is when there's no soft landing. There was grass below with a rough circle of damp earth where the grass had been worn away by the pounding of countless training jumps.

Suppressing my fear I jumped as instructed. The ground was harder than I'd expected, what with the rain earlier. I guess after thousands of feet landing on it, the dirt had become as hard as concrete.

After the landing practice Al called us all together.

"Looks like the weather isn't going to cooperate today. Those of you who don't want to wait and see if it clears up enough to jump today, can come back next week to jump." We all looked at each other as if to say "You want to stay?"

Small clusters of people whispered amongst themselves. I could see reluctant nods and thankful smiles spread throughout the class. I wondered how many would be saying their farewells and wishing us good luck.

"I think we're going to come back when the weather's better," said a tall man, holding hands with his much shorter wife. "Good Luck," he added shaking our hands, then heading quickly for their car.

"We're going to come back next week too," said the father of the Jamaican family of five. When all the good byes were said there were 10 of us left.

Two of the ten had been on a jump before and were back for more. This time they were jumping from 4800 feet, 2000 feet higher than we were. They'd been boasting about it all day.

Al looked us over, "So you're the brave ones, eh?" We all chuckled with excitement and embarrassed pride. "Well, if you have to use the toilet, now's a good time," he added, pointing to a row of blue chemical toilets better known as Porto Potties or Johnny on the Spot. The kind you find on any construction site or at an outdoor rock concert. Four of them stood next to the nearby wire fence. Approaching the nearest one, I could smell its nauseating ammonia and feces contents.

There was no immediate need to go, but I figured I'd better try. Who knew how my body was going to react when forced from the plane at 2800 feet.

Envisioning myself plummeting through the sky was enough to evacuate my lazy bowels and ½ full bladder. I walked from the stinky toilet with a smile on my face.

We gathered by the wind sock after the toilet. It wasn't sticking straight out any longer, but flapped angrily instead.

"Looks like we're going to jump today after all," said Al.

"Any questions before we board the planes?"

"Can I be first?" asked Pete without hesitation.

Damn, I wanted to be first.

"Second," I called out a heartbeat after Pete.

"Sure guys, any other questions?" No one said a word. They'd be content with whatever jumping order Al put them in.

"Okay then, let's get aboard," called Al walking towards the planes taxiing to a stop at the end of the dirt runway.

The ten of us glanced at each other and exchanged excited smiles. This was the last chance to back out and walk away. Once we were in the plane it would be too late.

"You five, come with me in this plane, the rest of you go with Bob here," said Al waving a hand at the handsome man stepping from the second plane. Bob gave a mock salute to Al. I noticed the two veteran jumpers went with Bob.

"Okay, board the plane in the reverse order you're going to jump. I'm going to give your harnesses a last check as you get aboard. I'll also be hooking a tether to your parachute so it'll open automatically once you've jumped. It can be a little overwhelming the first time and we don't want you to forget to pull your rip chord," he chuckled. We didn't.

The plane was a small twin engine model. The doorway we were to jump through was only four feet high and three feet wide. I noticed there wasn't a door.

Inside was cramped, no seats and barely enough room for the six of us to crouch with our parachute packs. Al crouched by the door making small talk with Pete and I until the engines roared and we started bumping along the runway. It got frighteningly noisy and rough before the wheels lifted from the ground, then everything including our stomachs smoothed right out. We were airborne.

Pete's eyes were wide with fear and adrenaline. He'd never been in a plane before, let alone jumped from one. This was the thrill of a lifetime for him and no small thrill for me either.

We soared higher and higher, then banked to the left. Pete couldn't wipe the smile from his face. It took about five minutes to reach twenty eight hundred feet.

"You ready?" asked Al grinning Pete. He nodded and gave the thumbs up.

"Good, sit right here with your legs out the door. Put your left hand here and your right hand here. That'll help you push yourself out," yelled Al, patting the silver metal sides of the door. Pete shuffled forward and sat in the tiny doorway with his legs out the door and only his ass inside the plane. He put his hands either side of the door and Al gave him a last piece of advice.

"Try to spread eagle as soon as you leave the plane. You ready?"

"Yeah," Pete screamed over the wind howling in through the doorway.

"Then GO!" yelled Al, and Pete was gone. Like he'd been sucked out of the plane.

I stuck my head out the door dying to see what had happened to Pete. There, far below and behind the plane was Pete spread eagled and spinning slowly like a snowflake. "Perfect jump," yelled Al in my ear.

The tether snapped on it's ring next to my head and I watched Pete's chute burst open. A second later he was hidden from sight by the all too close, tail of the plane.

"Your turn," yelled Al slapping my shoulder.

I smiled back at him and tried to swallow, but my mouth had been blow dried by the wind. When I grabbed the cold metal doorframe my hands slipped, my palms were moist with nervous sweat. I quickly wiped them on my pant legs and sat. As soon as my legs were out the door they were driven back towards the tail by the wind. After all, we were traveling at almost one hundred and sixty mph., against the wind. I had to hold tight to the sides of the door just to keep myself from being sucked out.

There was only a second to admire the view, but I could see for at least a hundred miles. Farms and forests for as far as the eye could see. Roads segmented the farms and there was Pete's chute drifting down, a speck of white against the green of the ground far below. He disappeared behind the tail wing of our plane not six feet from me.

"Man that tail wing sure looks close. Anybody ever get hit in the head when they jumped?" I yelled nervously.

"Naw, the second you're out of the plane you'll drop like a stone," Al said and smiled.

"How reassuring," I called over my shoulder while staring at the threatening tail wing.

"You ready?" asked Al.

I nodded, but kept looking out the door. "Okay GO!"

I froze. It's not natural to throw yourself from a perfectly good plane. I had a successful business, a hot Jamaican girlfriend, a loving family, and I was controlling my Diabetes and had a whole lifetime ahead of me. So why was I doing this again? Oh yeah, for the experience, the thrill, the rush, and while I could. Who knew what Diabetes would do to me later in life. I'd heard the stories of blindness, heart attacks and strokes. Seventeen years of near death reactions had already taught me to savor all the adventures and opportunities that came my way. This was just the most extreme adventure I'd ever tried. All this went through my mind in a single heart beat.

Then I leaned forward and hurled myself out of the plane. All my senses screamed "Ahhhhhh!" at once.

I was falling, fast, and spinning on an odd axis, because of my big feet. I saw the ground, then the plane, then the ground, then the plane again.

An incredible yank stopped my spinning and the chute noisily unfurled above me, jolting me again. It felt like I'd come to a complete mid-air stop.

The first thing that struck me, besides the fact that the tail wing hadn't, and I lived on, was the silence. After the roar of the plane engine and the wind screaming past the open door, all I could hear now was the distant drone of the plane far above me.

Remembering my earlier training I looked up for my steering toggles. They were dangling just in front of and above my shoulders. Grabbing them easily I reefed on the right one until it touched my right ankle. This maneuver swung me out beyond the edge of my chute, allowing me a three hundred and sixty degree view of the countryside. We'd been told to do this to get our bearings. Recalling the aerial photos we'd passed around in class, I quickly located the airstrip, barn and house.

I started pulling on the toggles to steer myself towards the target at the end of the airstrip. Al had advised us to land as close as possible. "That way you won't have as far to drag your chutes back to the barn after landing. The crackling sound of the radio strapped to my chest startled me.

"Jumper two, jumper two, left toggle," said the tinny voice.

I knew he was talking to me, so I pulled the left toggle to my waist and sailed left. From several hundreds of feet up the trees reminded me of blades of grass. The whole landscape below appeared more colorful and vibrant. This was as close to actual flying as I would ever get. It was magnificent.

Below and ahead of me, I saw Pete landing half way down the airstrip. His chute slowly and silently collapsed in front of him. I watched as his tiny figure jumped up and down before the wind caught his chute and dragged him off his feet. The radio voice drew my attention away from Pete and focused it back on where *I* was going.

After a series of left and right tugs on the toggles I was getting close to the ground. Looking between my feet, I watched the earth rush up to meet me, remembering at the last possible second, to look at the horizon when landing. My head shot up just before my toes touched the ground. I landed correctly, but hard. Rolling to the right my legs came up together in a splendid arc that ended with them both slamming into the ground. Pain shot through my knees.

Before I knew what was happening the wind had caught my chute and inflated it, turning it into a giant sail. I was dragged roughly along the ground, faster and faster.

I quickly grabbed the first cords I could lay my hands on and started hauling them towards me in a desperate attempt to close one side of the chute, thereby deflating it. I was dragged another thirty feet before succeeding.

I lay there a moment and caught my breath. Then I got up, took off my parachute harness and gathered my chute into a manageable pile, proudly carrying it down the airfield towards the barn.

Walking down the airstrip I kept looking back to check on the other Jumpers' progress, and make sure they weren't about to land on me. I watched the two bragging second timers land farthest from the target and laughed.

Then high overhead I heard a woman's voice screaming, "Ohhh, boy, oh boy, oh boy..."

It was tiny Marge, sailing by, high above my head. She was hauling on her toggles like a madman, one after the other, then both at the same time. She was completely out of control. I could hear the radio operator trying to give panic stricken Marge toggle instructions as she zipped past at what must have been a new club speed record.

She looked way too high to land anywhere near the target. Sure enough, a second later she flew over the target, then the end of the airstrip. She had to bend her knees, then raise them to her chest, to clear the busses. All the while yelling, "Oh boy, oh boy, oh boy...," faster and faster.

Marge finally came to a rolling stop a hundred yards away in the farmer's field next door. She lay there for a moment. Then all at once leapt up and started jumping up and down hooting and screaming with joy.

Pete had already dropped off his chute to the Riggers in the barn and was walking towards me with a big ass grin stretching from ear to ear. Suddenly his head tipped up slightly and his eyes widened. He silently mouthed, "Holy crap," and pointed up behind me.

I instinctively ducked and turned at the same time, not knowing what to expect. I mean, people were dropping out of the sky like flies.

Pete was pointing at Al who was coming in for a landing. He was still about sixty feet up but descending fast. He was using a colourful rectangular chute, the kind used in professional competitions.

I stood watching him sail by, the loose edges of his chute flapping and snapping in the wind. He swooped down and circled the target once. Then he made a series of quick short pulls on his toggles manoeuvring himself to hang right above the target bull's eye. His use of the toggles reminded me of a kid using the strings of a kite to make it dive and turn.

What he was doing looked impossible. He was facing into the wind and moving forward. He should have been blown away, but the way he handled that chute was awesome.

We stared up at him hovering there, 20 feet above the bull's eye for a good 5 seconds, looking down on either side, picking his spot. I looked around and saw that everyone else on the ground was staring up in disbelief. Then Al deftly tugged at his toggles and started drifting down, side to side, like a leaf falling from a tree. He was moving against the wind when he touched down, but both feet landed right on the bull's eye's red center and he came to a running stop. No crouched knees and rolling to one side for him. I have to admit I was envious of his parachuting prowess, but still applauded loudly with everyone else.

Pete turned to me and with a big grin said, "Did you see that? It was beautiful." I nodded and at the same time we said, "I want one of those next time." We laughed and watched the last few Jumpers from the second plane land without incident. Then I took my parachute to the Riggers in the barn.

Stepping out of the barn door I noticed two things. First I had the same big ass grin on my face that I'd seen spread across Pete's face moments earlier. The second thing was all the Jumpers standing around the radio operators table. It was set up under a huge white tent, on the edge of the airstrip.

Joining them we acknowledged each other with a nod, and big ass grins spread across our faces. There was also a twinkle in their eyes and I knew I had that twinkle too. You could feel it. We'd all overcome our fear of death, done something few in the world had done and survived. It confirmed, for me anyway, that I have value, perhaps even purpose. That the path I was on was right, my choices, good.

Al wore the same smile and had the same twinkle in his eye as he said, "Congratulations everyone, you made it." We all chuckled. "You were a great group. I'm proud to present you with your First Jump certificates." He called out the names in alphabetical order. Pete and I received our First Jump certificates like they were University Diplomas.

We each bought one of the T shirts we'd seen on display earlier in the house. All the way home comparing exciting stories of our jumps, swearing we'd do it again soon. I can't speak for Pete, but I never again felt the urge to hurl myself from a plane.

My First Jump certificate is framed and hangs on my office wall. I hung it there to remind me that Diabetics can do anything, but they should do it while they're able. Plus, remembering my first jump always puts a big ass smile on my face and a twinkle in my eye.

Chapter 8
Liquid Gold

Thursday

Have you ever run out of Maple Syrup? My wife Suzi told me we were syrupless, after bringing me a plate of hot, golden brown pancakes the size of Frisbees and plopping down a half empty jar of raspberry jam. I despise raspberry jam. "We should make our own syrup," I grumbled for the hundredth time, but instead of saying, "Oh wouldn't that be nice," like she had ninety nine times before, Suzi exclaimed, "What a great idea, ya think we can?"

"Sure, all ya gotta do is boil sap to make syrup," I blurted.

As the words passed my lips, a nagging doubt awoke and whispered, "Are you sure?"

Of course I wasn't sure. I'd never made maple syrup before in my life. But that didn't stop my ego from boasting, "Any monkey can boil sap," just begging Karma to send someone to smack my pompous ass with a humility stick.

That's when the phone rang. I knew Karma was behind the call before Suzi picked up the phone. It was Jerry my best friend. Coincidentally the proud owner of a humility stick with my name carved into it. Last week he'd called threatening to come up from the city for a short visit. This was more likely a cancelation than a confirmation call. You see, Jerry loves city life, the crowded sidewalks, flashing signs, countless restaurants and garish night clubs. He thinks of Huntsville as a pioneer village where fast food means you hit a deer with your pickup.

Suzi and Jerry chit chatted about health and weather, but avoided the reason for the call.

Suddenly Suzi exclaimed, "David's making maple syrup this weekend. Are you still coming up?"

I knew what he'd say, "Watching sap boil? Naw, I just watched some eggs boil and the thrill is gone. I'm gonna pass."

Suzi covered the mouthpiece with her hand, "Jerry says, don't start without him. He's dying to see how it's done."

"Me too," I whispered under my breath, but gave the thumbs up smiling. Karma chuckled while Suzi made the final arrangements, said good-bye and came back to the table. "Jerry says he's coming up Saturday. As usual he's not sure when, but before dinner for sure," she said, happily spreading jam on her pancakes.

"Excellent," I said with reservation. The tiniest mishap or mistake and he'd torment me with the stories whenever we got together with friends, or at parties, heck he'd tell strangers in bars just for a laugh. He'd get three sheets to the wind, pull out my humility stick and say, "Hey Davy, remember the time you made maple syrup and burned a hole the size of your head in the bottom of Suzi's favorite pot! Remember that? Eh? Eh?" Smack, smack, smack….

I had just two days to learn the basics and make a batch of maple syrup before Jerry arrived.

My nagging doubt stood up, cleared its throat, and said, "What's the plan?"

Plan? There was no plan. I'd been hoping that by cobbling together all my memories of maple syrup a plan would emerge. It's embarrassing to admit how incomplete my memories were. I didn't even know what a sugar maple looked like. Hitting the library or surfing the net would take all day and wouldn't give me the practical knowledge I needed right now. The clock was ticking.

Time to talk to an expert…time to talk to Bob.

Our neighbors Bob and Michelle own & operate Maple Bluff Farms, which produces maple syrup on a commercial scale. After breakfast I headed straight over. They greeted me warmly in French as I stepped from my car. I replied with a few practiced French phrases then switched to English to better beg for their help. They did help me, up off my knees, and even got me to stop crying by taking me on a tour of their Sugar Shack and offering equipment to get started.

"We ave eight tousand trees tapped," boasted Michelle.

"Eight hundred have buckets we still empty by hand," added Bob, "How many you need?"

"Six," I replied.

They laughed all the way to their Sugar Shack

I expected their sugar shack to be a rustic cabin in the woods behind their detached garage. Instead we walked right up to their garage and Bob swung up the big door. A cloud of warm sweet steam enveloped us. As it dissipated I saw their gigantic stainless steel cooker glistening in the morning sun. It stood twenty feet long, six wide, and eight tall. Three adjustable smoke stacks rose through the roof. In its belly three roaring wood fires heated three huge pans of sap. Swirling columns of steam danced above the golden surface before being drawn up the stacks. The sap in the closest pan was medium amber. *That's the color I'm gonna make my syrup,* I decided.

Bob answered my questions about boiling times and temperatures, identifying and tapping trees, when the season started and finished. At the end of the tour Bob gave me buckets, lids and a handful of what looked like silver cigar tubes.

"What are these," I asked examining one.

"Spiles," he said, like it was obvious.

"Ah," I said not wanting to look stupid. I'd google spiles later.

Bob saw my vacant stare adding, "Stick em in a hole and hang a bucket on it."

I drove home, anxious to tap my first tree. Visions of my own maple syrup empire dancing like sugar plums through my head. Stepping from the car I identified six sugar maples growing just sixty feet from my front door.

This is gonna be easy, I thought, but my nagging doubt taunted, "Jinx."

Shoving superstitious doubts aside, I dashed to the basement for a hammer and drill, but not just any drill. I wanted the whole pioneer experience and dug up the antique hand crank drill my father left me. It was a massive, six pound, rusty iron beast, eighteen inches long with cracked wooden handles. I had to spray the cogs with WD 40 oil before the handle would turn. I put the hammer and drill in the buckets then headed for the trees.

The snow around the trees was three feet deep with a thin crust. Tucking the buckets under one arm, I cautiously stepped up onto it. The crust squeaked & squealed under my boot heel, but held my weight. Testing each step, I moved towards the first tree.

Luck was on my side, or Karma was setting me up, I couldn't tell which, but I made it to the first tree without incident. I drilled a two inch deep hole at shoulder height. It took five minutes, and the effort made the muscles in my arms burn. I put the drill in the top bucket and pulled out the hammer and a spile.

Worrying the crust would collapse beneath me with each blow I tapped the spile into the hole, then separated a bucket and looped the handle over its exposed end. The handle slid right off. The bucket bounced and clattered across the snow to a stop several feet away. Sap began dripping from the spile.

Karma giggled.

I'd done something wrong, but what? After examining the other spiles, I noticed one end had a groove for the buckets' handle. I'd put the spile in backwards.

Karma chuckled in my ear while I pried the spile loose and hammered it back in correctly. This time the handle stayed firmly in place. Instantly drops of sap began hitting the bottom of the bucket, making a repetitive plink, plink, plink sound, literally the sweet sound of success. I'd tapped my first tree. My maple syrup empire was born. I attached the lid, closing it to keep rain, bugs, and twigs out.

Having had enough of the pioneer experience, I grabbed the old drill and raced to the basement, returning with a cordless drill in hand. I tapped the other five maples in ten minutes. Closing the last lid, I stopped to listen. Encircling me was the, plink, plink, plinking of sap dripping into six buckets, each with its own rhythm and tone. I lifted the lid of the first bucket and peeked inside. A quarter inch of clear sap already covered the bottom. At this rate the buckets would be full by tonight.

I carried the drill and hammer back to the house whistling Frank Sinatra's "I did it my way", but thinking, *Screw you nagging doubt.*

That afternoon the wind picked up and by dinner it was raining steadily. Before it got too dark, Suzi went to check the buckets. She was gone a long time. I was about to go check on her when the wind blew her through the front door, soaked from head to toe with a look of frustrated disappointment on her face. "The buckets were full of water, so I dumped them out," she stated.

"What, all of them?" I was stunned by the loss.

"Yeah, the wind must have blown the lids up and the rain in."

With Herculean effort I held my tongue, but my nagging doubt licked a finger and marked an invisible scoreboard, saying, "One day down, one to go."

Friday

I went with Suzi to check the buckets in the morning. Crossing the driveway she said, "Looks like a foot of snow melted overnight. Spring's coming." I didn't have the heart to tell her, but according to Bob the warm overnight temperatures meant the sap would stop running.

It also meant the snow no longer had a crust and we sank in up to our knees. Wading to the first tree I said, "Note to self, buy snowshoes for next year."
At the first tree, Suzi said, "How'd the bucket get up there?"

All six buckets, which hung shoulder high yesterday, now hung forehead high, an unforeseen effect of fast melting snow. While I explained my embarrassing short sightedness to Suzi, Karma slapped it's knee and guffawed behind my back.

Lowering the bucket we looked inside. It was full. I stopped Suzi from emptying it with a quick explanation. We lugged the sloshing buckets to our front porch. Last night at Canadian Tire I'd paid $12.00 for three propane bottles, $10.00 for a cooking adaptor, $5.00 for filter paper and $25.00 for a forty litre stainless steel cooking pot, because forty litres of sap makes one litre of syrup according to Bob.

The oversized pot sitting atop the propane bottle & adaptor looked like an elephant sitting on a bottle rocket. Remembering Bob's commercial cooker with its three 100 litre pans of fire heated sap, I felt a twinge of cooker envy. Jerry was bound to make a disparaging comment about buying the right equipment next time.

I knelt down to light the burner, pausing to savour the moment, lit match in hand. I was about to take another step towards independence. No more expensive store bought syrup. No more artificial table syrup. No more *raspberry jam.*

A breeze blew out the match, and the next one, but I managed to touch the third match to the burner and it popped to life. "Just a matter of time now," I thought, smiling.

An hour later, the sap had only boiled down a quarter inch. At this rate it would take till Sunday night to finish. Jerry would have come and gone before then. Bob had said, "A gentle boil is best," but I needed to move things along, so I did what anyone would do... I turned up the heat. When Suzi and I came back a couple of minutes later the sap was boiling violently.

"Is it supposed to boil that fast?" she asked.

"The faster, the better, don't worry I'll turn it down near the end."

"Well be careful you don't caramelize it."

"What does, "caramelize," mean?"

"Burn with style," she said heading back inside to make lunch.

Sixty minutes later the sap had dropped another whole inch. An hour after that the first bottle of propane ran out. I checked the level several times throughout the day and noticed the lower the level, the faster it dropped. With about 10 litres left in the pot, the second bottle of propane ran out.

Canadian Tire was closing soon, but I decided not to risk leaving the boiling syrup this close to success. I crossed my fingers hoping the third bottle would be enough to finish the job.

With only a couple of inches boiling away at the bottom of the pot, I ran into a wee problem. I knew the cooking was minutes from completion, but I also knew my bladder would explode if I waited another second.

I dashed to the bathroom, but forgot to turn down the heat.

When I got back, a thick column of grey smoke was billowing from the pot accompanied by the sound of crumpling cellophane. The air was rank with the stench of burnt sugar. Grabbing the handles I swung the pot off the burner and into the nearby snowbank. I'll never forget the loud, "fussssh," sound as a geyser of steam shot up, fogging my glasses. I staggered back and wiped off my glasses with my scarf. Waving aside the smoke and steam with both hands, I peered inside the pot.

There was no bubbling syrup, just a smouldering lump of shiny black slag fused to the bottom of the pot. Pulling the pot from its snow crater I examined the bottom, praying there wasn't a hole the size of my head.

The pot was intact. Scorched black inside and out, but it could boil another batch after a good scouring.

"Suzi," I called through the open front door, hoping she'd do the scouring.

"Is it done?" she called back from inside, excited anticipation in her voice.

How could I face her with this disaster then ask her to clean it up. Oh what the hell, it was worth a try.

I brought the still smoldering pot into the kitchen, head slightly bowed, eyes down cast.

"Wha, wha, what happened?" she exclaimed staring in horror at the failure in my hands like it was a dead baby.

"I swear, I only took my eyes off it for a second," I said with as much humility as I could muster. Karma fell to the floor laughing and kicking its feet in delight.

"Well I'm not cleaning up this mess," Suzi stated, scowling at the black lump in our new pot.

I worked late into the night scrubbing and scouring that pot back into usefulness. All the while my nagging doubt kept repeating, "Any monkey can boil sap, any monkey can boil sap..." I didn't sleep much that night, thinking about today's dismal failure and what tomorrow would bring...Jerry.

Saturday

The snow had all but vanished, leaving behind shallow puddles scattered across my driveway. Buckets, which just two days ago had been shoulder height, were now so high I could barely reach them, and they were overflowing.

By the time I'd lowered, lugged and emptied the third bucket into the cooking pot, I was soaked to the skin. I decided to get the second batch going, before I showered. The burner hissed to life, but when I struck the match, it went silent. The last propane bottle was empty.

I zipped to Canadian Tire only to find the price of propane had skyrocketed overnight. Three bottles now cost $15.00. "Next year I'm building a wood fire to boil sap," I promised the uninterested cashier as I paid for my six bottles of propane.

Back home I replaced the empty propane bottle, lit the burner and sat the ½ full pot on top. It was ten in the morning. I figured I had about 6 hours before Jerry arrived. The crunching sound of car tires on gravel made me spin around. Jerry's green TR8, or as he calls it, 'The Land Rocket', was racing up our driveway, music blaring and horn honking.

He skidded to a gravel spraying stop, threw it into park, revved it twice, sending wildlife for cover, before killing the engine. The eerie silence that followed was like being in the eye of a hurricane. Then the tiny car's door flew open and Jerry stepped out.

When I saw his expensive leather shoes hit the gravel I knew he wouldn't be lugging any sloppy buckets of sap anywhere. Heck, with his leather bomber jacket, designer jeans, and buttoned dress shirt he didn't even look dressed for today's cooler weather.

"Hey nature boy, how ya doin?" he called out, removing his sunglasses with one hand and tossing them on the front dash. Instead of answering, "Fine Jerry, and you?" I said, "What are you doing here?" "I came to help you make Maple Syrup, remember?" Grabbing his overnight bag from the trunk he added, "Maybe I'll take home a few litres for my restaurant." *A few litres,* I thought, *What an optimist.*

After greeting Suzi and unpacking, we went to collect the remaining sap. Jerry tiptoed across the moist forest floor and stood under the first bucket. "Why'd you hang them so high?" he asked reaching up, unable to touch the bucket's bottom. I explained about the rapid snow melt while Karma retrieved the humility stick from the back seat of Jerry`s car and handed it to him. As I lowered, lugged and emptied the buckets, Jerry followed behind with his stick, insisting there had to be a better, faster, and cleaner way to get sap to the cooker than mine. Smack, smack, smack.

I took a quick shower then lit the burner. Ten minutes later the sap was boiling, gently this time.

"That's it? It just boils?" asked Jerry stifling a yawn. I nodded.

"Boy this is gonna be fun, got any beer?" he added.

We sat there on the front porch, drinking beer and shooting the breeze while the sap boiled. Every now and again he'd look at the pot and ask a question. "How long do you have to boil it?"

"About ten hours," I replied, but my nagging doubt said, "How would you know?"

Jerry exclaimed, "Ten hours?!" like he'd been given an unjust life sentence in prison. I got him another beer. One beer later, glancing into the pot again, he asked, "When do you add the color?"
Was he pulling my leg? Raising an eyebrow I said, "You don't add color, it gets darker as it boils down."
Later Jerry came back from a bathroom break with two beers in hand and a puzzled look on his face.
"How do you make it thicker? Do you add corn starch?" he asked, handing me a beer while peering into the pot.
"The longer it boils the thicker it gets," I said, twisting the cap off my beer.
My nagging doubt repeated, "How would you know?"
After our next beer Jerry asked a question I'll never forget.
"Do you have to plant new trees every year?"

I looked him straight in the eye to see if he was joking, drunk, or just plain stupid. I mean honestly, did he think trees grew from seed to 40' tall each spring shooting up through the snow like crocuses? Or that we drained the sap from them each year then chopped them into campsite firewood? Next thing you know he'd be asking if we tapped sugar free trees to make diet syrup. He had to be pulling my leg. I mean if he wasn't... well if he wasn't, I was going to take that humility stick and give him a concussion with it.

Then I had an epiphany. Jerry wasn't joking, or irretrievably stupid. He was a typical child of the city, born and raised, completely disconnected from the natural world. A Cidiot. In his mind, nature was what man conquered, or at least tamed, to survive. The 40' trees that lined his city's streets arrived ready to plant with root balls wrapped in burlap. The part where those trees grew from seed to full height was missing. When city trees are badly damaged, or die, they're cut up, carted away, and replaced by an adult tree, and higher taxes.

Suddenly the idea bulb above my head flickered to life. No matter how bad this batch of syrup turned out, Jerry couldn't humiliate me with its stories. His one *dumb* question would put that humility stick in my hands for quite a while. I reached over and took it from Jerry the new village idiot, before answering him.

"No Jerry, they're not annuals." I knew full well he didn't know the difference between an annual and a perennial, or that the terms referred to flowers not trees. Smack, smack, smack.

Jerry smiled and said, "Ahh," as if my answer had made perfect sense. I smiled back, turned and smacked Karma upside the head, then stepped over its unconscious form and went inside to get us another beer.

By six o'clock, the syrup was done. There wasn't much, just three small jam jars full. To celebrate our tiny victory Suzi made French toast, sausages and bacon for dinner, with a fresh fruit salad for dessert. I took extra insulin before we ate, just so I could pour syrup over everything. I don't know if it was because I'd made it myself, or what, but my taste buds had never known such pleasure. The syrup was perfect. Suzi and Jerry agreed, mouthful after mouthful. So I pulled my confidence pistol from its shoulder holster and shot my nagging doubt right between its beady little eyes.

The End
(until next year)

www.ingramcontent.com/pod-product-compliance
Lightning Source LLC
Chambersburg PA
CBHW062008280526
45787CB00005B/2017